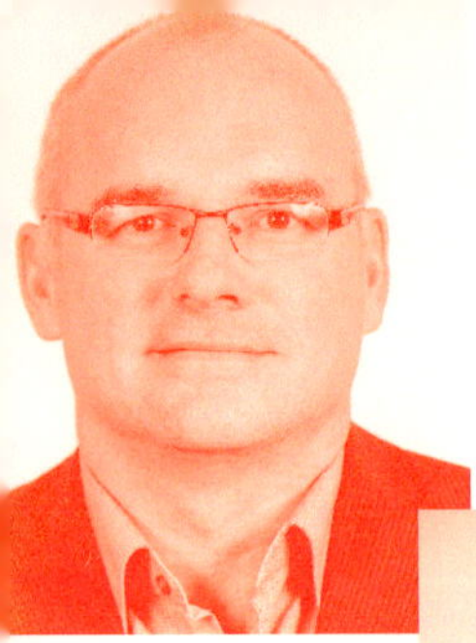
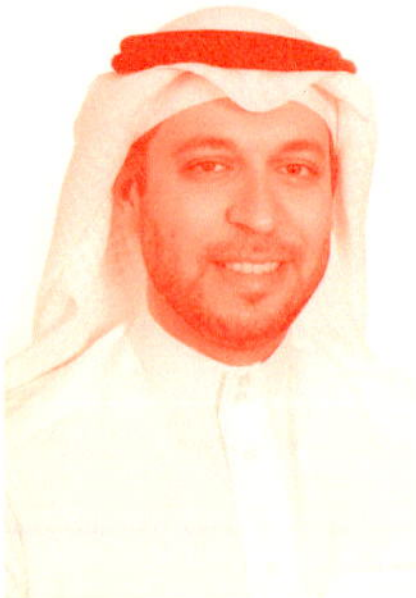
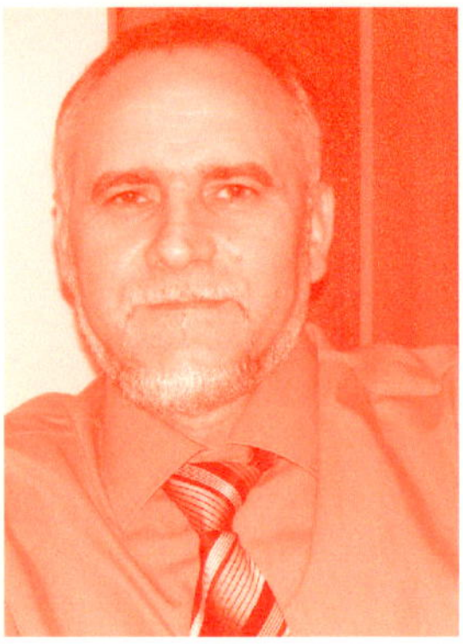
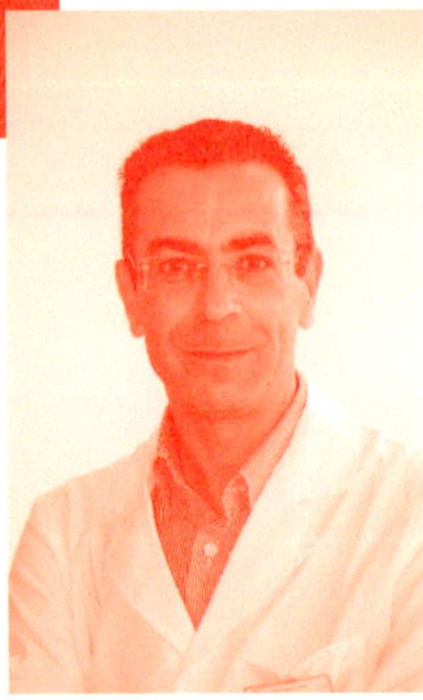
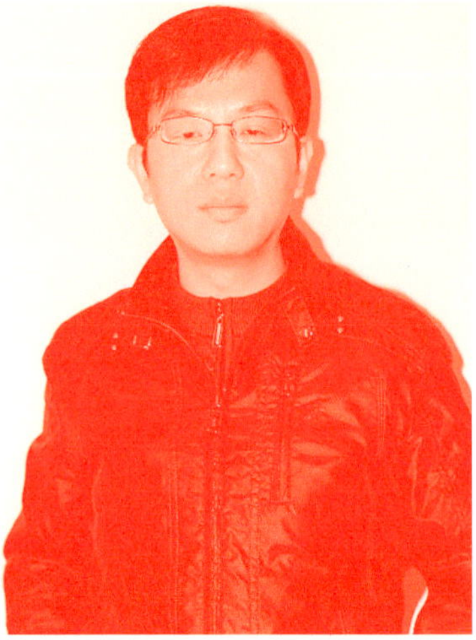
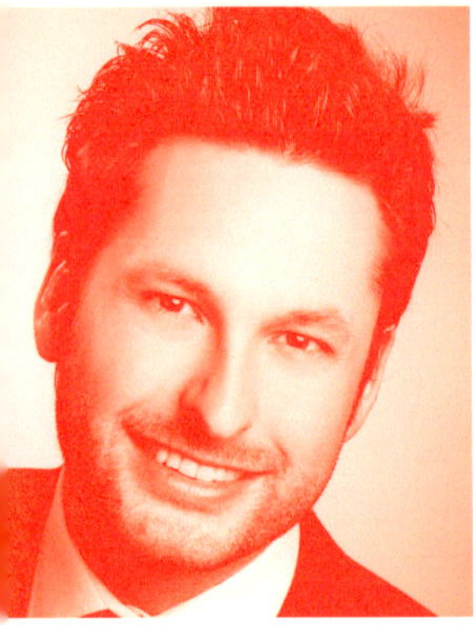
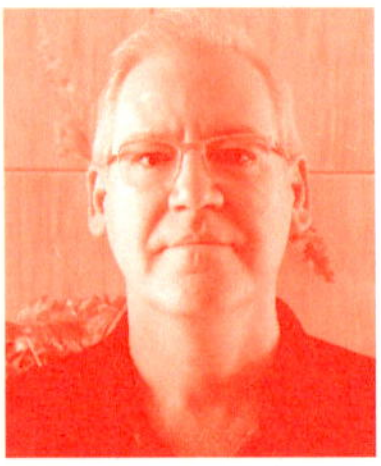

IntechOpen

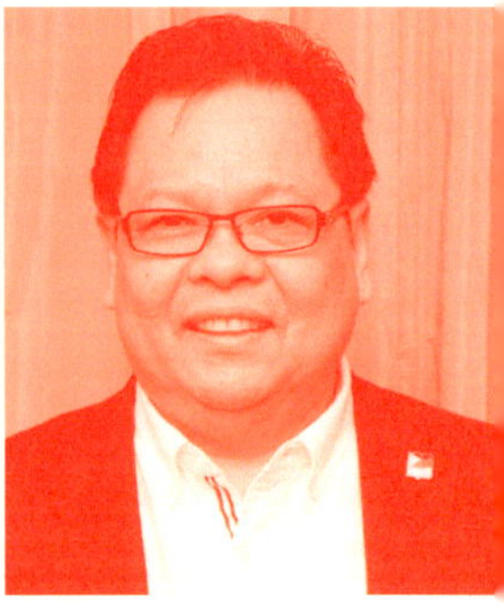
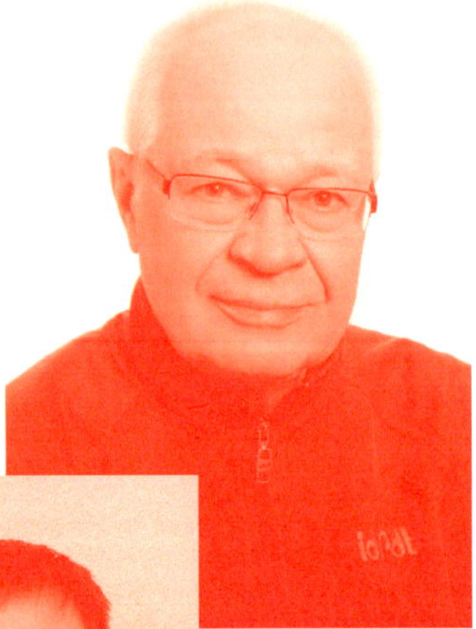
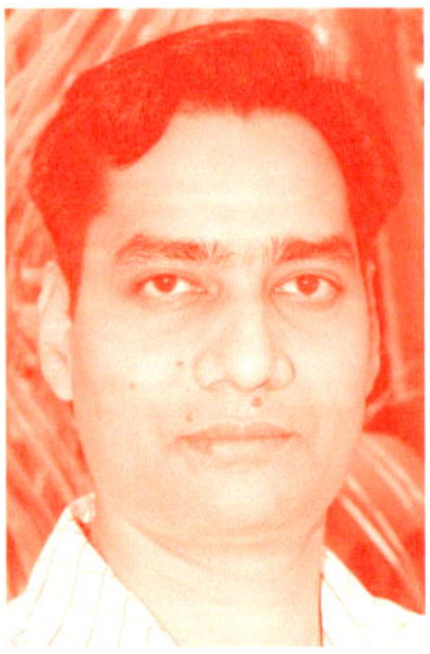
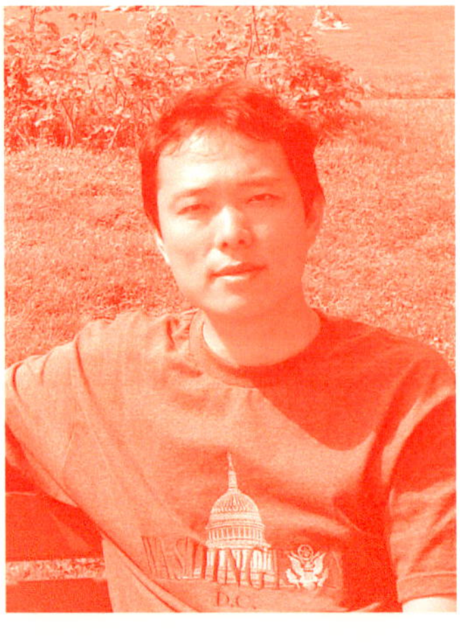
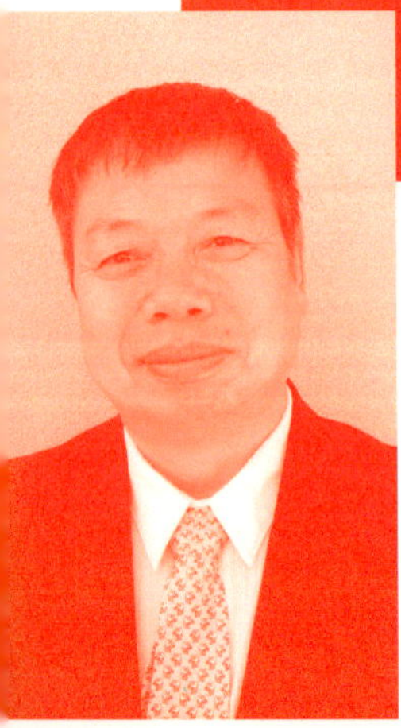
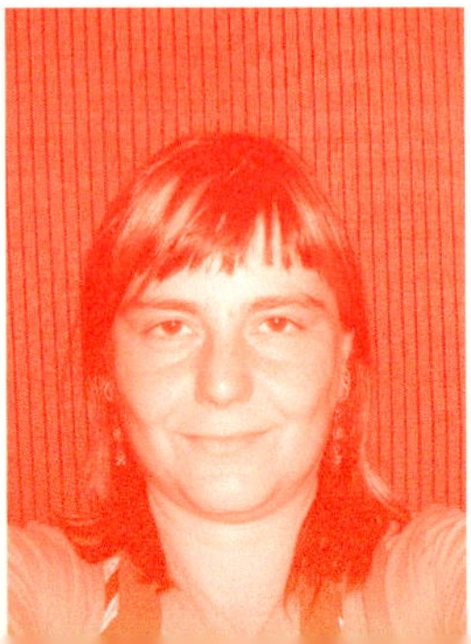

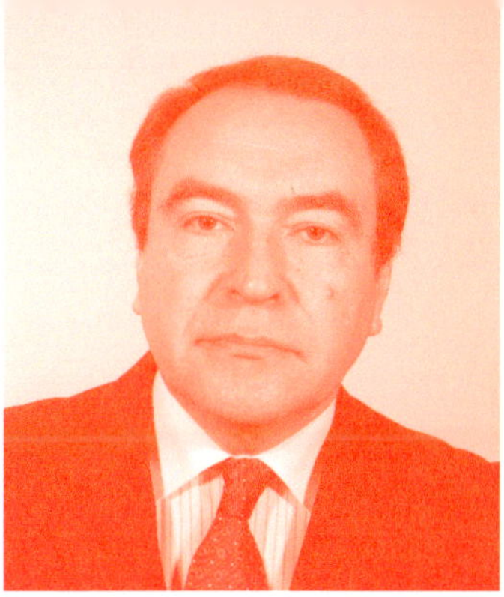

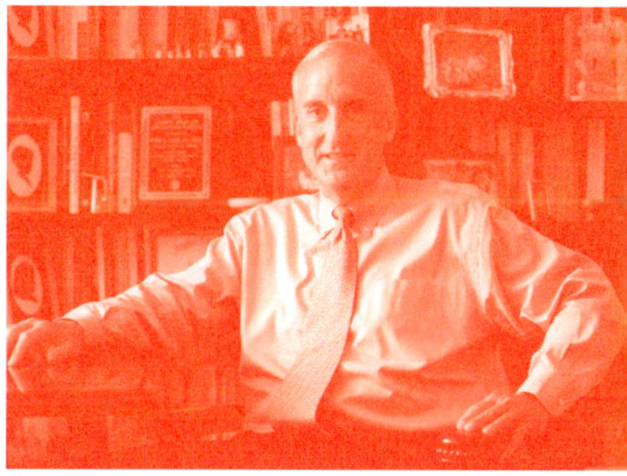

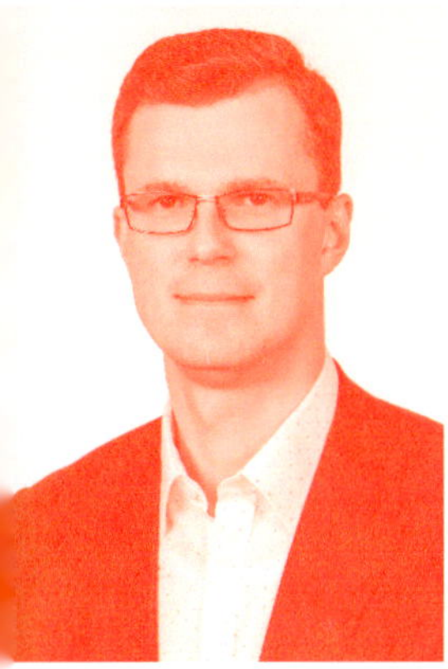

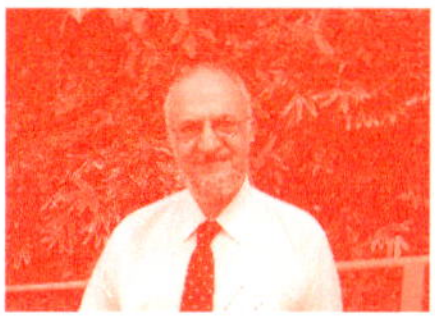

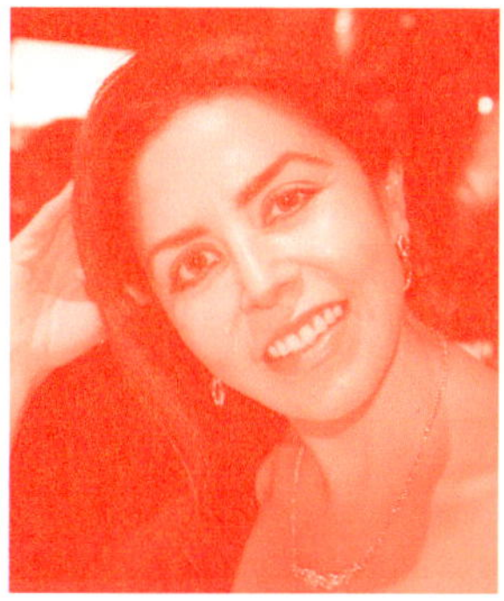

Supporting open minds since 2005

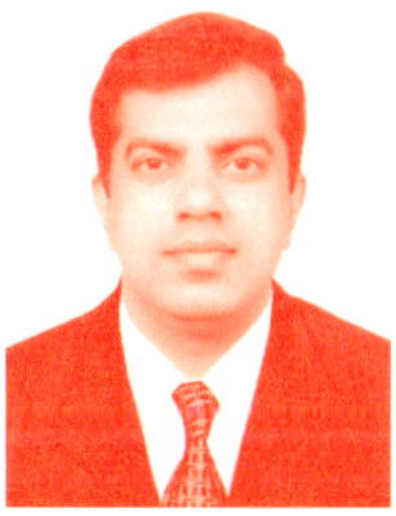

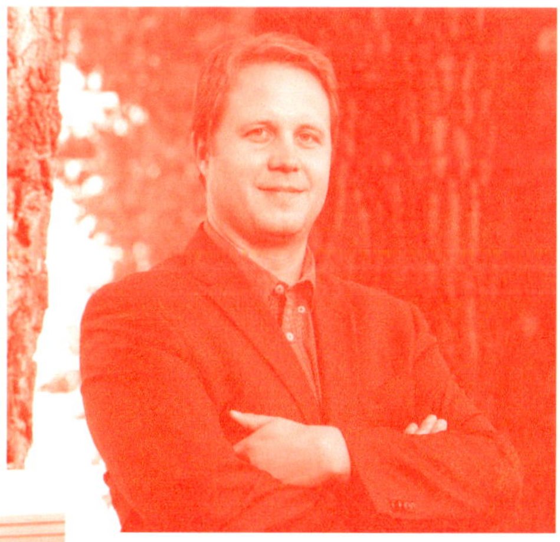

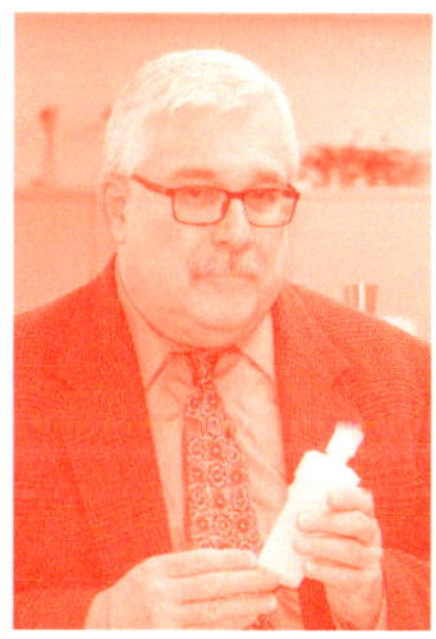

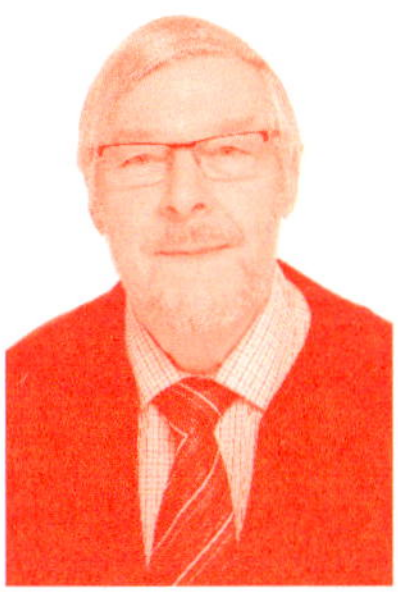

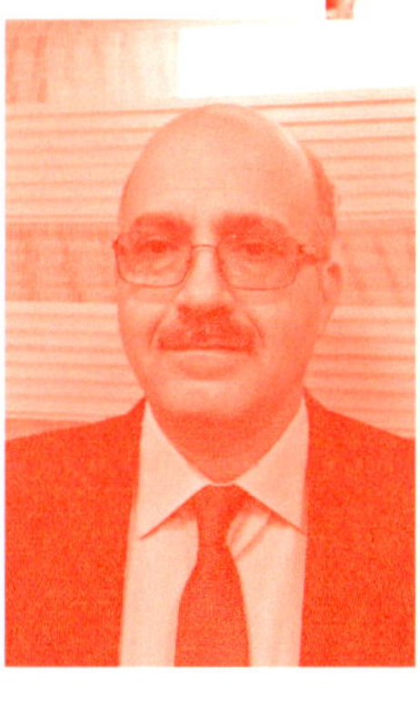

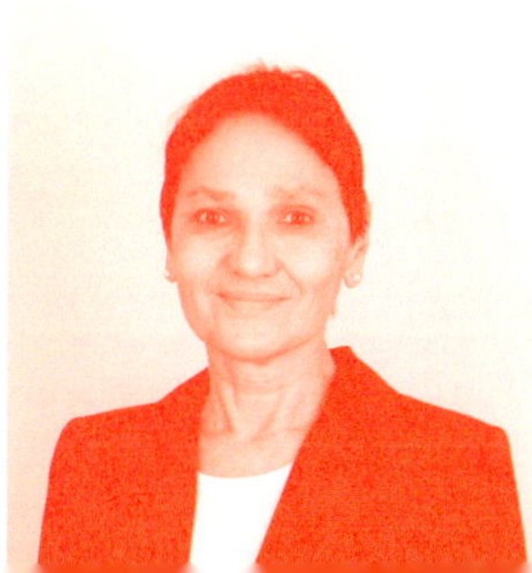

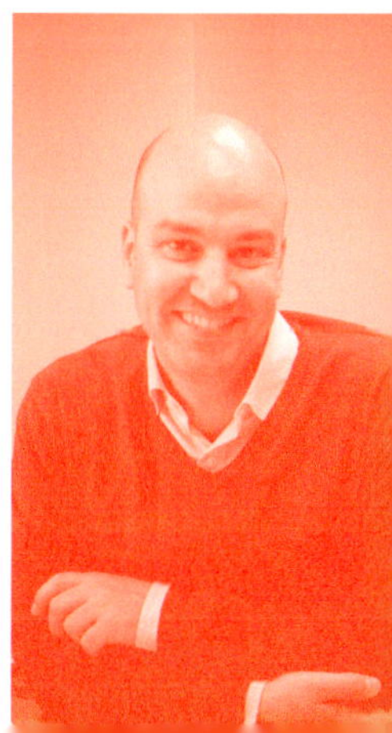

Mechanical Ventilation
http://dx.doi.org/10.5772/intechopen.95746
Edited by Jessica Lovich-Sapola, Jonathan A. Alter and Maureen Harders

Contributors
Iuri Christmann Christmann Wawrzeniak, Karolinny Borinelli De Aquino Moura, Eder Chaves Pacheco, Amal Francis Sam, Anil Yogendra Yadav, Pavol Pobeha, Jessica Lovich-Sapola, Jonathan Alan Alter, Maureen Harders, Pierre Singer, Liran Statlender, Thierry Hernandez-Gilsoul, Jose De Jesus Vidal-Mayo, Alan Alexis Chacon-Corral, Carmen Silvia Valente Silvia Valente Barbas, Sergio Nogueira Nemer, Lauren F. Goodman

First published in London, United Kingdom, 2022 by IntechOpen
IntechOpen is the global imprint of INTECHOPEN LIMITED, registered in England and Wales, registration number: 11086078, 5 Princes Gate Court, London, SW7 2QJ, United Kingdom
Printed in Croatia

British Library Cataloguing-in-Publication Data
A catalogue record for this book is available from the British Library

Additional hard and PDF copies can be obtained from orders@intechopen.com

Mechanical Ventilation
Edited by Jessica Lovich-Sapola, Jonathan A. Alter and Maureen Harders
p. cm.
Print ISBN 978-1-83969-728-9
Online ISBN 978-1-83969-729-6
eBook (PDF) ISBN 978-1-83969-730-2

For EU product safety concerns:
IN TECH d.o.o., Prolaz Marije Krucifikse Kozulić 3, 51000 Rijeka, Croatia, info@intechopen.com or visit our website at intechopen.com.

Meet the editors

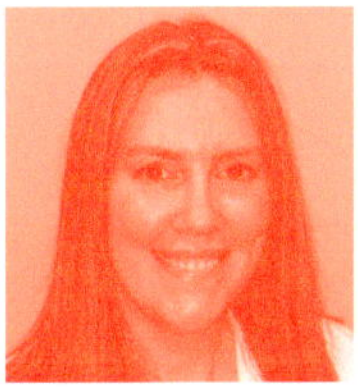

Jessica Lovich-Sapola is an associate professor at Case Western Reserve University School of Medicine (SOM), USA. Jessica completed her degrees MD at the Northeast Ohio Medical University (NEOMED) and MBA at Cleveland State University. She is a fellow of the American Society of Anesthesiologists (ASA). Jessica is a board-certified anesthesiologist at MetroHealth Medical Center, where she serves as president of the medical staff and associate director of anesthesia quality. Her academic focus is on trauma, burn, and regional anesthesia. She has authored five peer-reviewed articles, over 100 book chapters, and 18 abstracts presented at national meetings. She is also the editor of the 1st and 2nd editions of the book: *Anesthesia Oral Board Review: Knocking Out the Boards*. Jessica serves on committees for the Ohio Society of Anesthesiologists (OSA) and the Society for Ambulatory Anesthesia (SAMBA).

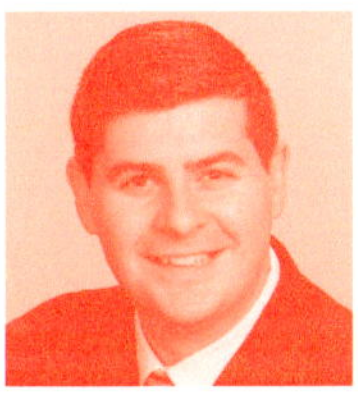

Jonathan Alter is an anesthesiologist at MetroHealth Medical Center in Cleveland, Ohio, assistant professor at Case Western Reserve University School of Medicine, and director of presurgical testing at MetroHealth Medical Center.

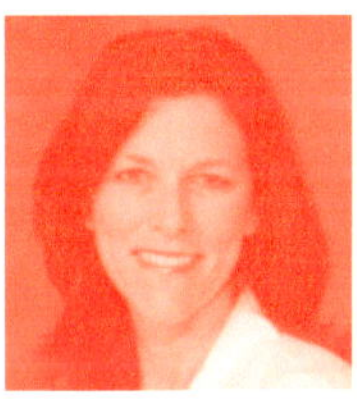

Maureen Harders is a board-certified anesthesiologist at MetroHealth Medical Center in Cleveland, Ohio, an assistant professor at Case Western Reserve University School of Medicine, director of anesthesia operations at MetroHealth Medical Center, director of anesthesia quality at MetroHealth Medical Center, and director of ambulatory anesthesia: outpatient surgery at Parma and level III trauma center at MetroHealth Medical Center.

Contents

Preface

Mechanical ventilation, ventilator management, and weaning from mechanical ventilation vary based on location within the hospital, the type of lung injury, and the medical condition of the patient. Understanding the types of lung injury and various methods of achieving ventilation expand the armamentarium of a practitioner and allow for the best management decisions to be made.

This book is a reference tool for the most up-to-date information on critical-care ventilation. It begins with the use of a high-flow nasal cannula (HFNC) and a detailed description of the advanced modes of ventilation. Once the types of ventilation are understood, they will then be applied to the ventilation approaches in different populations of patients: the trauma patients, the obese patients, and the patients under neurocritical care.

The final chapters contain a discussion of the mechanisms on how to wean from mechanical ventilation, how certain medical conditions affect the weaning process, and finally the approach to palliative withdrawal of mechanical ventilation.

This book is intended to give the reader a comprehensive overview of mechanical ventilation in the intensive-care unit and operating-room settings based on the most recent literature.

Jessica Lovich-Sapola, MD, MBA, FASA, Jonathan Alter, MD and Maureen Harders, MD
MetroHealth Medical Center,
Cleveland, Ohio, USA

Section 1

Modes of Ventilation

Chapter 1

High-Flow Nasal Cannula

Amal Francis Sam and Anil Yogendra Yadav

Abstract

Conventionally, oxygen is given at 4 to 6 L/min through nasal cannula for supplementation of oxygen. The FiO_2 achieved through this can be up to 0.4. Flows more than this can cause dryness to the nasal mucosa without much increase in the FiO_2. High-flow nasal cannula (HFNC) uses flow up to 60 L/min. Positive end-expiratory pressure is created in the nasopharynx and it is also conducted to the lower airways. Studies have shown HFNC improves washout of CO2 and decreases respiratory rate. Patient compliance also improves due to the comfort of the cannula compared to the non-invasive ventilation through a mask.

Keywords: non-invasive ventilation, high-flow nasal cannula, positive end-expiratory pressure, humidification

1. Introduction

Typically, respiratory support devices fit into three major categories: conventional oxygen delivery devices, non-invasive respiratory support, and invasive respiratory support. High-flow nasal cannula (HFNC) comes under a new category between conventional oxygen delivery device and non-invasive respiratory support. High-flow oxygen *via* non-rebreather mask can supplement oxygen at high concentration, provided the flow is around 10–15 L/min. At this rate, the medical gas is not humidified efficiently and this unwarmed and dry gas causes mask discomfort, and eye, oral, and nasal irritation [1]. Non-invasive ventilation is conventionally administered with a tight-sealing face mask, which might cause discomfort to the patient. Hence, it is associated with poor compliance when compared to other oxygen delivery systems. A device with better compliance with some added advantages of positive end-expiratory pressure (PEEP) and humidification would be a blessing to the patients and the caregivers.

In 1987, for the first time, oxygen therapy at a maximum flow rate of 20 L/min, with heated humidification system, was used in oxygen therapy for patients with bronchiectasis and cystic pulmonary fibrosis to promote the removal of lower respiratory tract secretions. It is still being extensively studied in respiratory distress syndrome, in apnea of prematurity in the neonate and pediatric units [2]. In adults, it has been used to treat acute respiratory failure, high-risk extubations in ICU, and many other clinical scenarios.

2. Mechanism

HFNC has an air/oxygen blender, which delivers the gas at desired FiO_2 regardless of the flow rate. The heated humidifier is an inline system and actively humidifies the inspiratory gas. Other conventional oxygen therapy (COT) devices mostly through bubble humidification deliver non-humidified or under-humidified gas to the patient. Additionally, the nasal cannula of HFNC differs from the conventionally used nasal prongs by being loose, larger, and softer, which improves tolerance (**Figure 1**).

2.1 Mucociliary clearance and humidification

Epithelial cells of the respiratory tract when exposed to dry gas for 4 to 8 h have been shown to have reduced function and increased inflammation. The mucociliary clearance was studied with saccharin transit times, and there was 40% delay in the transit when patients were supplemented with dry non-humidified or under-humidified oxygen. Hence, adequate humidification is vital in maintaining the functions of respiratory epithelial cells [3]. Breathing unwarmed dry gas can increase resistance and decrease pulmonary compliance as well [4]. This is also partly attributed to receptors in the nasal mucosa, which results in muscarinic receptors-mediated bronchoconstriction in the lower airways [5].

During spontaneous breathing of room air, humidification is actively done by the nasal mucosa and nasopharynx. As per Dalton's law, the warmer the gas, the more water vapor is held. In this process of heating, some energy expenditure occurs in the human body. Supplementation of heated and humidified air reduces energy expenditure and can reduce CO2 production and decrease oxygen consumption. This mechanism is also supported by the study in infants, which showed increased weight gain in patients treated with HFNC [6, 7].

2.2 Washout of dead space

About 30% of the tidal volume does not participate in gas exchange. This is due to the anatomical dead space from the nose to the terminal bronchiole. The volume of this dead space is fixed and when the tidal volume reduces, the proportion of dead space ventilation increases. The effect of this dead space is higher in shallow breathing in a patient with respiratory insufficiency. In acute respiratory distress syndrome (ARDS), this dead space ventilation can go above 60% above the tidal volume (i.e., $V_D/V_T \geq 0.6$) [8]. In a spontaneously breathing patient, HFNC

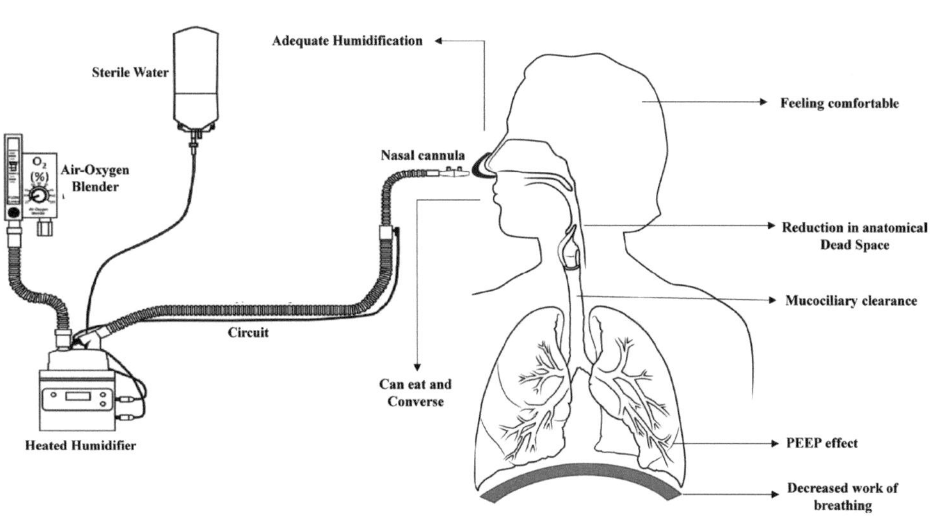

Figure 1.
Components and effects of HFNC.

washes out the exhaled gas in the nasopharynx and replaces this dead space with a lower CO2 and higher oxygen air mixture, and this oxygen-rich air is breathed in by the patient at the next cycle, which helps in washing out the CO2. It was evident by the reduction in minute ventilation at a constant arterial CO2 tension and pH, in the studies [9].

2.3 Patient acceptance

Non-invasive ventilation (NIV) has a low acceptance rate from the patient point of view due to the discomfort of tight-fitting mask and variable levels of humidification according to the type of humidification used. Studies have shown that HFNC is better tolerated than NIV [10]. Also, when compared with face mask (FM), oxygen supplementation with a bubble humidifier HFNC is shown to be better tolerated. In a study involving oxygen supplementation at 15 L/min through FM with bubble humidifier and HFNC, patients on HFNC had greater overall comfort level, lower dyspnea scores, and reduced mouth dryness [11].

In “do not intubate” scenario, there is no change in outcome observed between NIV and HFNC, but the patients who were on HFNC had better diet intake, who conversed until just before their death. People like to eat by themselves and to talk with their friends and family at the end of their life, and HFNC favored patients in these requirements [12].

2.4 Work of breathing

The peak inspiratory flow in patients with respiratory failure is around 60 L/min and HFNC can match this flow, when compared with COT devices, and hence helps in reducing the work of breathing during the inspiration. The reduction in work of breathing was also evident in the form of lower inspiratory esophageal pressure swing, better compliance ($V_t/\Delta Pes$), and lower PTP and PTP_{min} in HFNC group compared with face mask and oxygen [9].

2.5 PEEP effect

At higher flow rates through the nasal cannula, positive pressure is created in the nasopharynx. The effect of positive pressure is higher when the patient is breathing with the mouth closed as it creates a seal. Some amount of airway pressure is lost if the patient opens the mouth.

The mean pressure generated with flows between 10 and 15 L/min was 1.7 to 5.3 cm H_2O. Anatomical differences in the nares’ size and variability in the airway among the patients, varying leak around the bores of the HFNC, might have led to this wide variation in the pressure created in the airway [13]. The positive pressure created in the airway is maximum at the end of expiration. For each increase of 10 L/min of flow, there is an increase in mean airway pressure of 0.69 cm H_2O, in patients breathing with mouth closed. It decreases to 0.35 cm H_2O if the patient is breathing with mouth open [14]. These studies have measured the pressure changes by placing a catheter through the nasopharynx and placing the tip of the catheter at the level of uvula. Whether this pressure created in the nasopharynx is conducted down to the respiratory system is the next question. There is an increase in functional residual capacity when electrical impedance tomography is used to study the effect of HFNC. The pressure created in the nasopharynx by the high flow is transmitted down to the lower airways and there is an increase in the lung volume. The increase in lung volume is much homogenous in the prone position when compared to supine position. In the supine position, the expansion of lung is predominant in the ventral region [15].

3. Clinical use

3.1 Difficult intubation

In case of difficult intubation, HFNC can be given to patients as a method of pre-oxygenation and can be continued during induction, relaxation, and laryngoscopy. Clinicians should note that a jaw thrust is necessary to keep the airway in continuum with the nasopharynx. This method is called Trans-nasal Humidified Rapid-Insufflation Ventilatory Exchange (THRIVE), which has improved the apneic time up to 17 min with $PaCO_2$ levels around 60–75 mm Hg [16]. It is a potential alternative to high-flow intra-tracheal oxygen insufflation for apneic oxygenation. Patients could maintain oxygen saturations for a longer time during the apneic oxygenation and this could change the nature of difficult intubations from a hurried stop-start event to a smooth event.

3.2 Hypoxemia

The mechanisms of action of HFNC and its comfort make it a first-line oxygen delivery device for adult patients with hypoxemia. The beneficial effects of HFNC are evident by reduction in respiratory rate and improvement in oxygen saturation [17]. It not only improves the numbers in arterial blood gas, but also improves the patient clinically in terms of dyspnea score, supraclavicular retraction, and thoraco-abdominal asynchrony. All these benefits can be seen as early as 15–30 min [18]. When compared with COT devices, HFNC has shown to have reduced requirement of NIV for rescue [19].

However, the results were not the same in other studies. In a study involving patients presenting with respiratory failure to the emergency department, HFNC was not superior to COT devices in terms of escalation to mechanical ventilation, length of hospital stay, and 90-day mortality. Similar results were seen in FLORALI trial, except for reduced mortality at 90 days in patients treated with HFNC [20]. Authors attributed this benefit to degree of comfort, the heating and humidification of inspired gases, which prevented thick secretions, low levels of PEEP generated by a high gas flow rate, and reduction in dead space.

In a meta-analysis, authors concluded that, in hypoxemic patients with respiratory distress, HFNC was not better than COT devices in terms of mortality, but when compared with initiation of mechanical ventilation and escalation of therapy, HFNC was associated with risk reduction [21]. In immunocompromised patients with respiratory failure, HFNC was associated with reduction in the rate of intubation and mechanical ventilation when compared with the COT devices and NIV [22]. HFNC is also useful in treating patients with stable hypercapnic COPD and obstructive sleep apnea [23, 24].

3.3 Extubation in ICU

Extubation in intensive care unit is associated with 12–14% of re-intubation mostly within 72 h. NIV is advised in high-risk patients to prevent early re-intubation [25]. HFNC can be an alternative to NIV in patients with high risk of re-intubation. However, the results were contradictory. Compared with conventional oxygen delivery devices, HFNC has reduced the incidence of re-intubation in high-risk patients in few studies and it has not, in few other studies [26–29].

3.4 Postoperative management

In cardiothoracic postoperative patients, HFNC is equal to NIV in preventing postoperative pulmonary complications. Patients treated with HFNC and NIV had similar rates of treatment failure and mortality. But for the ease of nursing care and better acceptance from the patients, HFNC can be an alternative to NIV in postoperative cardiac surgeries [30]. In case of major abdominal surgeries, the incidence of hypoxemia in the postoperative period is 10–50% according to various studies. Pulmonary complications are due to loss of functional alveolar units because of de-recruitment and basal atelectasis. In this subset of postoperative patients, HFNC was inferior to NIV in preventing hypoxemia and in terms of length of stay [29].

3.5 Pediatrics

There is a lack of guidance of flow in the pediatric population. About 1–2 L/min, for less than 24 months, is advised and sometimes a flow of 0.5 L/min is used in neonates. Regarding cannula size for the pediatric patients, the manufacturers recommend that the cross-sectional area of the cannula should not be more than 50% of the cross-sectional area of the nares and the outer diameter of the cannula should not be more than two-thirds than that of the nares. Discrepancies in size might lead to unexpected elevations in airway pressure or excess air leak.

In optimum conditions, the pressure created by the HFNC is comparable to nasal CPAP. But with increasing leak, the pressure effect diminishes and varies between patients. A pressure release valve is necessary in neonatal HFNC as the flow is fixed and directly delivered to the infant, to prevent over distension and injury [31]. In a retrospective study involving premature infants with neonatal respiratory disease, there were no differences in incidence of bronchopulmonary dysplasia, and no difference in rate of infection and death. But more infants were intubated for failing early nasal CPAP compared with early HFNC [32]. In another study involving nasal CPAP and HFNC as a prophylaxis to prevent re-intubation in high-risk preterm infants, HFNC failed to maintain the extubation status of the preterm infants [33]. When compared with COT, HFNC has shown to reduce extubation failures in pediatric population [34].

In addition to respiratory failure, post-extubation, and pre-oxygenation, acute bronchiolitis is the main indication for HFNC in pediatric patients. In studies, there were no differences in length of stay, intubation rate, respiratory rate (RR), SpO_2, or adverse events in patients treated with HFNC versus COT devices and nasal CPAP groups. But treatment failure was higher in the HFNC group when compared with nasal CPAP group and lower in the HFNC group when compared with COT devices group [35]. In status asthmaticus, HFNC when compared with COT devices had better pCO_2 levels, pH, improvement in SpO2, and reduction in respiratory rate [36]. In children who do not tolerate CPAP for OSA, HFNC has proved to be a better alternative. In a study involving children not tolerating CPAP, use of HFNC has reduced obstructive apnea-hypopnea index by 9 events/h and desaturation episodes by 13 events/h on an average [37]. HFNC stands between COT devices and CPAP in bronchiolitis and for prophylaxis after extubation. Better designed, larger studies are needed for other indications and comparisons with other oxygen delivery and ventilating systems.

3.6 Initiation and titration

In a patient with acute respiratory distress, first the eligibility of the patient for non-invasive support is to be assessed. Whoever it does not fit in the criteria should be intubated to protect the upper airway and mechanical ventilated. Patients who can be given a trial of HFNC are started at 40 L/min flow, 100% FiO_2, and 31°C temperature. Temperature of 31°C is more comfortable to patients than temperature of 37°C. FiO_2 is titrated down for a SpO_2 target of 90%. Patient is assessed after 1–2 h and in case of respiratory rate > 35/min or the FiO_2 requirement is more than

45%; then, the flow is increased by 5–10 L/min. Once the maximum recommended flow of 60 L/min is reached, FiO_2 is gradually increased for the desired targets. The targets are SpO_2 just above 90% and respiratory rate less than 35/min (**Figure 2**).

In case of clinical improvement, first the FiO_2 is titrated down to 40–50%, and then, the flow is titrated down 5–10 L/min per session. The frequency at which the flow is adjusted depends on the clinical situation. Once the flow reaches less than 20 L/min, the patient can be weaned from HFNC and can be put on COT devices [38].

HFNC is being attributed to delay in intubation and studies have shown increased mortality in such situations. Failure of HFNC might cause delayed intubation and worse clinical outcomes in patients with respiratory failure [39]. Roca et al. derived an index to predict the success of HFNC in patients with respiratory failure and pneumonia. ROX (Respiratory rate – OXygenation) index with oxygenation as numerator (SpO_2/FiO_2 ratio) and respiratory rate as denominator is calculated after 12 h of initiation of HFNC therapy. A value less than 4.88 identified patients who will fail HFNC and require intubation (area under curve of 0.74; 95% CI, 0.64–0.84) [40]. This index was also externally validated, and their calculated cutoff was 3.85. A score of more than 4.88 suggests therapeutic success of HFNC and a score of less than 3.85 is suggestive of failure of HFNC and needs intubation as delayed intubation is associated with poor outcomes. There is a gray area between 3.85 and 4.88. In that case, ROX index to be calculated after 1–2 h and in case if it is increasing, then invasive mechanical ventilation is recommended (**Figure 3**).

3.7 Adverse effects

HFNC is more expensive than COT devices and that limits its widespread use. When compared with COT devices and NIV, administration of HFNC is considered as an aerosol-generating procedure. This might put the health care workers at risk and in case of a communicable disease, this will be an additional burden during an epidemic or a pandemic. The aerosol dispersion can be up to 17 cm from the patient, with the use of HFNC at 60 L/min. This dispersion is higher than the simple face mask delivering oxygen at 6 L/min, but it is lesser than the devices that deliver higher flows such as non-rebreathing face mask (24 cm) and venturi mask (39 cm) [41, 42]. Clinician should make sure the fit and seal of the HFNC is satisfactory, or else the lateral spread of aerosol can be as high as 60 cm in case the interface is loose. In another study involving patients with bacterial pneumonia, who were either on HFNC or on face mask, with settle plates at 0.4 and 1.5 meters from

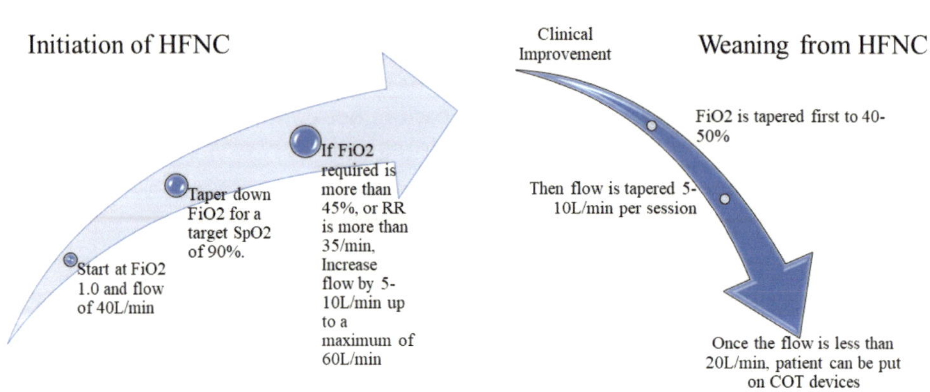

Figure 2.
Initiation and titration of HFNC. FiO2—Fraction of inspired oxygen. SpO2—oxygen saturation in blood. RR—respiratory rate. COT—Conventional oxygen therapy (Adapted from Ischaki et al. [38]).

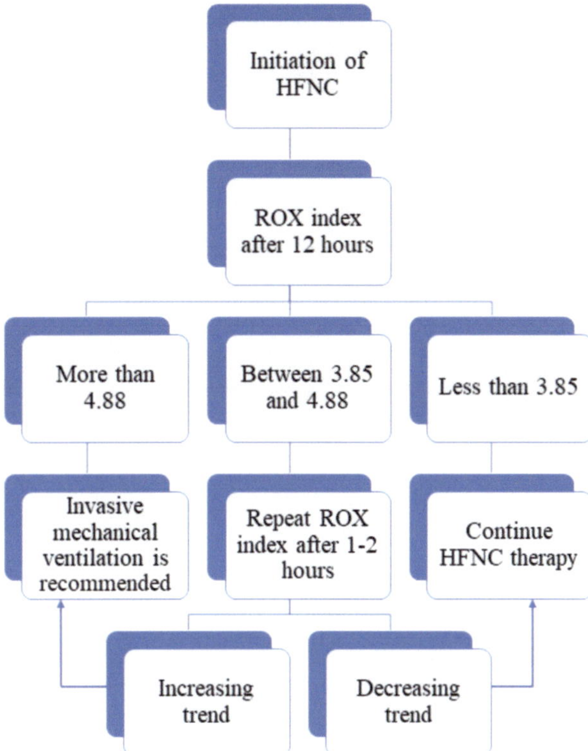

Figure 3.
Utility of ROX index. ROX—Respiratory rate-OXygenation (adapted from Roca and Messika et al. [40]).

patients, there was no significant difference in bacterial counts in the air sample between HFNC and face mask [43]. Even though studies do not establish transmission of disease through HFNC, there is uncertainty and fear of aerosol dispersion [44, 45]. Addition of a surgical mask over the HFNC can prevent aerosolization, which is not possible in case of oxygen face masks [46].

Similar to NIV, HFNC also has the potential for delaying intubation when clinically indicated. Patients who got invasively ventilated after 48 h of NIV had higher mortality than those intubated and ventilated within 48-h therapy. Hence, early detection of NIV/HFNC failure is vital for optimum management [38].

One of the beneficial effects of HFNC is the positive pressure created in the airway, but that can be maximum up to 7 cm H_2O and there is loss of positive pressure if the patient opens the mouth [14]. When compared with COT devices, HFNC had higher PaO_2, but the effect was attributed to higher FiO_2 achieved as the PF ratio was unaffected. But when compared with HFNC, NIV not only had higher PaO_2, but also higher PF ratio, which was attributed to its higher PEEP effect. The peak inspiratory flow generated by patients with respiratory failure is around 60 L/min, which can increase further, when there can be entrapment of room air, which will affect the FiO_2 achieved, whereas the FiO_2 delivered to the patient using NIV can reach 100% with proper seal and the higher flow demand of the patient is also matched by the ventilator.

3.8 Complications

Prolonged use of HFNC may lead to abdominal distension, aspiration, and barotrauma, although the risk of barotrauma is much less as compared with non-invasive or mechanical ventilation. A well-known complication of HFNC is barotrauma such as air trapping, pneumothorax, and pneumomediastinum. The equipment is costlier and involves more technology and accessories than conventional nasal cannula. There is a learning curve for the caregivers but that is usually quickly achieved.

3.9 Contraindications

HFNC is contraindicated in patients who are unresponsive or agitated and patients at risk of aspiration. HFNC will be of limited use in patients with airway obstruction due to tumors. Facial anomalies, recent or past facial surgery, or facial trauma might hinder the use of HFNC. It is better avoided in patients with upper airway surgery to avoid the theoretical risk of venous thromboembolism due to the high pressure during its use.

4. Conclusion

HFNC lies in between conventional oxygen delivery devices and NIV. HFNC has been used to treat hypoxemic respiratory failure, cardiogenic pulmonary edema, and post-extubation prophylaxis to decrease pulmonary complications, and in high-risk extubations. However, most of the studies addressing these are of low quality to draw conclusions and strong recommendations. HFNC can be of useful value in a setup where there is continuous monitoring of patients.

Author details

Amal Francis Sam* and Anil Yogendra Yadav
Institute of Liver and Biliary Sciences, New Delhi, India

*Address all correspondence to: amalfsam@gmail.com

References

[1] Tanaka D, inventor; Cordis Corp, assignee. Long term oxygen therapy system. United States patent US 7,086, 398. 2006

[2] Manley BJ, Dold SK, Davis PG, Roehr CC. High-flow nasal cannulae for respiratory support of preterm infants: A review of the evidence. Neonatology. 2012;**102**(4):300-308

[3] Chidekel A, Zhu Y, Wang J, Mosko JJ, Rodriguez E, Shaffer TH. The effects of gas humidification with high-flow nasal cannula on cultured human airway epithelial cells. Pulmonary Medicine. 2012;**2012**:380686. DOI: 10.1155/2012/380686

[4] Greenspan JS, Wolfson MR, Shaffer TH. Airway responsiveness to low inspired gas temperature in preterm neonates. The Journal of Pediatrics. 1991;**118**(3):443-445

[5] Fontanari P, Burnet H, Zattara-Hartmann MC, Jammes Y. Changes in airway resistance induced by nasal inhalation of cold dry, dry, or moist air in normal individuals. Journal of Applied Physiology. 1996;**81**(4):1739-1743

[6] Dysart K, Miller TL, Wolfson MR, Shaffer TH. Research in high flow therapy: mechanisms of action. Respiratory Medicine. 2009;**103**(10):1400-1405

[7] Holleman-Duray D, Kaupie D, Weiss MG. Heated humidified high-flow nasal cannula: Use and a neonatal early extubation protocol. Journal of Perinatology. 2007;**27**(12):776-781

[8] Kallet RH, Zhuo H, Liu KD, Calfee CS, Matthay MA. The association between physiologic dead-space fraction and mortality in subjects with ARDS enrolled in a prospective multi-center clinical trial. Respiratory Care. 2014;**59**(11):1611-1618. DOI: 10.4187/respcare.02593

[9] Mauri T, Turrini C, Eronia N, Grasselli G, Volta CA, Bellani G, et al. Physiologic effects of high-flow nasal cannula in acute hypoxemic respiratory failure. American Journal of Respiratory and Critical Care Medicine. 2017;**195**(9):1207-1215

[10] Frat JP, Brugiere B, Ragot S, Chatellier D, Veinstein A, Goudet V, et al. Sequential application of oxygen therapy via high-flow nasal cannula and noninvasive ventilation in acute respiratory failure: an observational pilot study. Respiratory Care. 2015;**60**(2):170-178

[11] Roca O, Riera J, Torres F, Masclans JR. High-flow oxygen therapy in acute respiratory failure. Respiratory Care. 2010;**55**(4):408-413

[12] Koyauchi T, Hasegawa H, Kanata K, Kakutani T, Amano Y, Ozawa Y, et al. Efficacy and tolerability of high-flow nasal cannula oxygen therapy for hypoxemic respiratory failure in patients with interstitial lung disease with do-not-intubate orders: A retrospective single-center study. Respiration. 2018;**96**(4):323-329

[13] Parke R, McGuinness S, Eccleston M. Nasal high-flow therapy delivers low level positive airway pressure. British Journal of Anaesthesia. 2009;**103**(6):886-890

[14] Parke RL, Eccleston ML, McGuinness SP. The effects of flow on airway pressure during nasal high-flow oxygen therapy. Respiratory Care. 2011;**56**(8):1151-1155

[15] Riera J, Pérez P, Cortés J, Roca O, Masclans JR, Rello J. Effect of high-flow nasal cannula and body position on end-expiratory lung volume: A cohort

study using electrical impedance tomography. Respiratory Care. 2013; **58**(4):589-596

[16] Patel A, Nouraei SR. Transnasal humidified rapid-insufflation ventilatory exchange (thrive): A physiological method of increasing apnoea time in patients with difficult airways. Anaesthesia. 2015;**70**(3): 323-329

[17] Lenglet H, Sztrymf B, Leroy C, Brun P, Dreyfuss D, Ricard JD. Humidified high flow nasal oxygen during respiratory failure in the emergency department: Feasibility and efficacy. Respiratory Care. 2012;**57**(11): 1873-1878

[18] Sztrymf B, Messika J, Bertrand F, Hurel D, Leon R, Dreyfuss D, et al. Beneficial effects of humidified high flow nasal oxygen in critical care patients: A prospective pilot study. Intensive Care Medicine. 2011;**37**(11): 1780-1786

[19] Parke RL, McGuinness SP, Eccleston ML. A preliminary randomized controlled trial to assess effectiveness of nasal high-flow oxygen in intensive care patients. Respiratory Care. 2011;**56**(3):265-270

[20] Frat JP, Thille AW, Mercat A, Girault C, Ragot S, Perbet S, et al. High-flow oxygen through nasal cannula in acute hypoxemic respiratory failure. The New England Journal of Medicine. 2015;**372**(23):2185-2196

[21] Rochwerg B, Granton D, Wang DX, Helviz Y, Einav S, Frat JP, et al. High flow nasal cannula compared with conventional oxygen therapy for acute hypoxemic respiratory failure: a systematic review and meta-analysis. Intensive Care Medicine. 2019;**45**(5): 563-572

[22] Cheng LC, Chang SP, Wang JJ, Hsiao SY, Lai CC, Chao CM. The impact of high-flow nasal cannula on the outcome of immunocompromised patients with acute respiratory failure: A systematic review and meta-analysis. Medicina. 2019;**55**(10):693

[23] Nagata K, Kikuchi T, Horie T, Shiraki A, Kitajima T, Kadowaki T, et al. Domiciliary high-flow nasal cannula oxygen therapy for patients with stable hypercapnic chronic obstructive pulmonary disease. A multicenter randomized crossover trial. Annals of the American Thoracic Society. 2018; **15**:432-439

[24] McGinley BM, Patil SP, Kirkness JP, Smith PL, Schwartz AR, Schneider H. A nasal cannula can be used to treat obstructive sleep apnea. American Journal of Respiratory and Critical Care Medicine. 2007;**176**:194-200

[25] Schmidt GA, Girard TD, Kress JP, Morris PE, Ouellette DR, Alhazzani W, et al. Liberation from mechanical ventilation in critically ill adults: Executive summary of an official American College of Chest Physicians/ American Thoracic Society clinical practice guideline. Chest. 2017;**151**(1): 160-165

[26] Hernández G, Vaquero C, Colinas L, Cuena R, González P, Canabal A, et al. Effect of postextubation high-flow nasal cannula vs noninvasive ventilation on reintubation and postextubation respiratory failure in high-risk patients: A randomized clinical trial. JAMA. 2016;**316**(15):1565-1574

[27] Maggiore SM, Idone FA, Vaschetto R, Festa R, Cataldo A, Antonicelli F, et al. Nasal high-flow versus Venturi mask oxygen therapy after extubation. Effects on oxygenation, comfort, and clinical outcome. American Journal of Respiratory and Critical Care Medicine. 2014;**190**(3):282-288

[28] Futier E, Paugam-Burtz C, Godet T, Khopy-Ear L, Rozencwajg S, Delay J-M,

et al. Effect of early postextubation high-flow nasal cannula vs conventional oxygen therapy on hypoxaemia in patients after major abdominal surgery: A French multicentre randomised controlled trial (OPERA). Intensive Care Medicine. 2016;**42**(12):1888-1898

[29] Parke R, McGuinness S, Dixon R, Jull A. Open-label, phase II study of routine high-flow nasal oxygen therapy in cardiac surgical patients. British Journal of Anaesthesia. 2013;**111**(6): 925-931

[30] Stéphan F, Barrucand B, Petit P, Rézaiguia-Delclaux S, Médard A, Delannoy B, et al. High-flow nasal oxygen vs noninvasive positive airway pressure in hypoxemic patients after cardiothoracic surgery: a randomized clinical trial. Jama. 2015;**313**(23): 2331-2339

[31] Lampland AL, Plumm B, Meyers PA, Worwa CT, Mammel MC. Observational study of humidified high-flow nasal cannula compared with nasal continuous positive airway pressure. The Journal of pediatrics. 2009;**154**(2):177-182

[32] Shoemaker MT, Pierce MR, Yoder BA, DiGeronimo RJ. High flow nasal cannula versus nasal CPAP for neonatal respiratory disease: A retrospective study. Journal of Perinatology. 2007;**27**(2):85-91

[33] Campbell DM, Shah PS, Shah V, Kelly EN. Nasal continuous positive airway pressure from high flow cannula versus infant flow for preterm infants. Journal of Perinatology. 2006;**26**(9): 546-549

[34] Akyıldız B, Öztürk S, Ülgen-Tekerek N, Doğanay S, Görkem SB. Comparison between high-flow nasal oxygen cannula and conventional oxygen therapy after extubation in pediatric intensive care unit. Turkish Journal of Pediatrics. 2018;**60**(2)

[35] Lin J, Zhang Y, Xiong L, Liu S, Gong C, Dai J. High-flow nasal cannula therapy for children with bronchiolitis: A systematic review and meta-analysis. Archives of Disease in Childhood. 2019;**104**(6):564-576

[36] Baudin F, Buisson A, Vanel B, Massenavette B, Pouyau R, Javouhey E. Nasal high flow in management of children with status asthmaticus: A retrospective observational study. Annals of Intensive Care. 2017;7(1):1-9

[37] Hawkins S, Huston S, Campbell K, Halbower A. High-flow, heated, humidified air via nasal cannula treats CPAP-intolerant children with obstructive sleep apnea. Journal of Clinical Sleep Medicine. 2017;**13**(8): 981-989

[38] Ischaki E, Pantazopoulos I, Zakynthinos S. Nasal high flow therapy: A novel treatment rather than a more expensive oxygen device. European Respiratory Review. 2017;26(145).

[39] Kang BJ, Koh Y, Lim CM, Huh JW, Baek S, Han M, et al. Failure of high-flow nasal cannula therapy may delay intubation and increase mortality. Intensive Care Medicine. 2015;**41**(4): 623-632

[40] Roca O, Messika J, Caralt B, García-de-Acilu M, Sztrymf B, Ricard JD, et al. Predicting success of high-flow nasal cannula in pneumonia patients with hypoxemic respiratory failure: The utility of the ROX index. Journal of Critical Care. 2016;**35**:200-205

[41] Hui DS, Chow BK, Lo T, Tsang OT, Ko FW, Ng SS, et al. Exhaled air dispersion during high-flow nasal cannula therapy versus CPAP via different masks. European Respiratory Journal. 2019;**53**(4)

[42] Ip M, Tang JW, Hui DS, Wong AL, Chan MT, Joynt GM, et al. Airflow and droplet spreading around oxygen masks:

a simulation model for infection control research. American Journal of Infection Control. 2007;**35**(10):684-689

[43] Leung CC, Joynt GM, Gomersall CD, Wong WT, Lee A, Ling L, et al. Comparison of high-flow nasal cannula versus oxygen face mask for environmental bacterial contamination in critically ill pneumonia patients: A randomized controlled crossover trial. Journal of Hospital Infection. 2019;**101**(1):84-87

[44] Li J, Fink JB, Ehrmann S. High-flow nasal cannula for COVID-19 patients: Low risk of bio-aerosol dispersion. European Respiratory Journal. 2020; **55**(5):2000892

[45] Loh NW, Tan Y, Taculod J, Gorospe B, Teope AS, Somani J, et al. The impact of high-flow nasal cannula (HFNC) on coughing distance: Implications on its use during the novel coronavirus disease outbreak. Canadian Journal of Anaesthesia. 2020;**67**:893-894

[46] Hui DS, Chow BK, Chu L, Ng SS, Lee N, Gin T, et al. Exhaled air dispersion during coughing with and without wearing a surgical or N95 mask. PLoS One. 2012;**7**(12):e50845

Chapter 2

Advanced Modes of Mechanical Ventilation

Carmen Silvia Valente Barbas and Sergio Nogueira Nemer

Abstract

Advanced modes of mechanical ventilation emerged from the need for better control of the ventilator by the patient, the possibility of respiratory mechanics and respiratory drive monitoring in assisted modes and a better patient-ventilator synchrony. Volume-assured pressure support ventilation (VAPSV) has the advantage of the variable of flow pressure support ventilation (PSV) assuring tidal volume in each respiratory cycle. Proportional assist ventilation plus (PAV+) delivers assistance in proportion of inspiratory efforts while monitoring work of breathing, respiratory compliance, resistance and auto-PEEP, improving patient-ventilator asynchrony. Neurally adjusted ventilatory assist ventilation (NAVA) provides diaphragmatic electroactivity information and a better inspiratory and expiratory patient-ventilator synchrony. Adaptative support ventilation (ASV) assures a pre-set minute ventilation adjusting Pressure Support according to respiratory rate. Intellivent-ASV adds SpO2 and PETCO2 monitoring to adjust minute ventilation and PEEP/FIO2 according to lung pathology. Smart-Care ventilation provides an algorithm that decreases PSV according to patients tidal volume, respiratory rate and ETCO2 according to lung pathology and performs a spontaneous breathing trial indicating the redness for extubation. Clinical indications of advanced modes are to improve patient-ventilator synchrony and provide better respiratory monitoring in the assisted modes of mechanical ventilation.

Keywords: new modes of mechanical ventilation, VAPSV, PAV+, NAVA, ASV, Smart Care®

1. Introduction

When patients with acute respiratory failure recovery from the respiratory insufficiency, they are transitioned to assisted modes of ventilation to start the weaning process. The most common assisted modes are volume assisted ventilation in which the ventilator delivers the same tidal volume during every inspiration, and Pressure support ventilation (PSV) in which the ventilator delivers the same delta pressure assistance during every inspiration. The fixed deliver tidal volume or pressure assistance are the main reason for the occurrence of patient-ventilator asynchrony in these modes of ventilation. In PSV, the inspiratory flow is variable resulting in less asynchrony than in volume assisted ventilation, however asynchrony can still be present in cases of patients with obstructive lung disease and ineffective efforts or under assistance with insufficient tidal volume, can also occur especially in patients with low respiratory system compliance or high respiratory resistance. In these cases, the patients' tidal volume cannot be guaranteed and the patient can generate a huge inspiratory effort that is often under detected. During PSV, the same assistance is independent of the patient's demand, allowing under or over-assistance and the occurrence of patient-ventilator asynchrony [1]. The advanced modes of mechanical ventilation emerged from the need of greater control of the ventilator by the patient, the possibility of better synchrony and monitoring of the respiratory mechanics during the assisted modes of mechanical ventilation [1].

2. Volume assured pressure support ventilation

Volume assured pressure support ventilation (VAPSV) is a dual mode of mechanical ventilation that associates pressure support ventilation to volume assisted ventilation. This combination optimizes the inspiratory flow, decreasing the patient's work of breathing while assuring the set tidal volume. Compared to volume assisted ventilation, VAPSV can decrease the patient's respiratory drive (a lower measure P0.1), the pressure -time product and the patient's work of breathing. This advanced mode of ventilation extends the benefits of PSV to unstable patients with acute respiratory failure, assuring a pre-set tidal volume (**Figure 1**) [1].

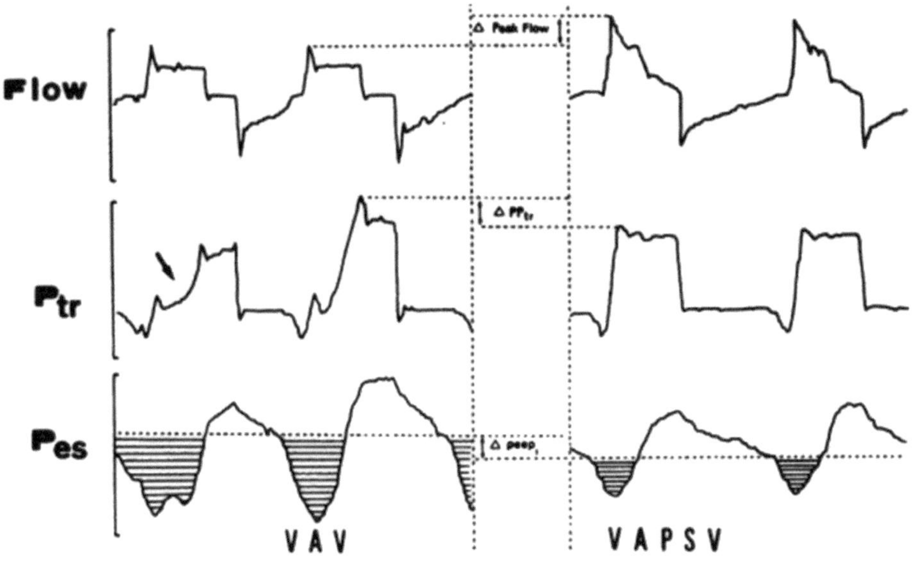

Figure 1.
Volume assisted ventilation (VAV) compared to volume assured pressure support ventilation (VAPSV): note the decrease of the esophageal pressure and the better inspiratory flow synchrony during VAPSV [1].

3. Proportional assist ventilation (PAV)

Proportional modes deliver assistance in proportion to the patient's demand, allowing variation of inspiratory pressure and avoiding diaphragm excessive loading and atrophy by disuse. Proportional assist ventilation (PAV) is a form of synchronized ventilator support in which the ventilator generates pressure in proportion to the instantaneous patient effort, or in proportion to flow and volume generated by the same [2–4]. Therefore, the ventilator allows at any time during inspiration, airway pressure in proportion to the pressure generated by inspiratory muscles (Pmus) and respiratory mechanics [4].

Initially described by Magdy Younes in 1992, PAV amplifies inspiratory efforts with the goal of the patient comfortably attain whatever ventilation and breathing pattern that the control system desires [2].

There is no target tidal volume, mandatory rate and airway pressure preset [5]. The ventilator is able to automatically adapt to changes in ventilatory demand of the patient. The pressure delivered by the ventilator follows the Pmus profile, usually with a progressive increase from the beginning of inspiration, with gradual pressurization, to the end of inspiration [4]. Maximal assistance is achieved until the end of inspiration [4].

Unlike PSV, in which a constant preset level of pressure assists each inspiration, regardless of the patient's inspiratory effort, PAV allows assistance proportional to the patient's demand, avoiding under-assistance or over-assistance [4], frequently observed during PSV. Under-assistance can induce respiratory distress and over-assistance can cause overdistension, and both may generate patient-ventilator asynchrony, that are associated with poor outcomes [5].

Therefore, PAV is designated for patients with stable respiratory drive, and can be used in any patient who is being ventilated under pressure support ventilation (PSV) or during weaning from mechanical ventilation [2, 6]. PAV is also designated to improve synchronism, while generating proportional assistance [2, 6].

3.1 How PAV works

PAV plus (PAV+) or Proportional Pressure Support (PPS) represent an upgrade to PAV [4] and are the clinically available versions of PAV.

During assisted ventilation, both the patient and ventilator contribute to the pressure required to overcome the elastic and resistive load during tidal breathing, according to the equation of motion [6]:

$$\mathrm{Pmus} + \mathrm{Pvent} = \mathrm{V}' \mathrm{x}\, \mathrm{R} + \mathrm{V}\, \mathrm{x}\, \mathrm{E} + \mathrm{P}_{\mathrm{EE}} \quad (1)$$

where Pmus is the pressure generated by respiratory muscles, Pvent is the pressure provided by the ventilator, V′ is the instantaneous flow, V is the volume, R and E are the resistance and elastance of the respiratory system respectively, and finally, P_{EE}, is the elastic recoil pressure at end-expiration [7].

During PAV+, the ventilator software calculates elastance or compliance of the respiratory system and airway resistance using a brief end-inspiratory occlusion performed randomly every four to ten breaths [7, 8]. During each end-inspiratory occlusion, a 300 ms pause allows the ventilator to measure compliance (Crs) or elastance of the respiratory system (Ers) [9] and airway resistance (Raw). Based on inspiratory effort and respiratory mechanics, the ventilator adjusts inspiratory pressure, according to the equation of motion. As patient demand changes, PAV can also change proportionally inspiratory pressure above positive end-expiratory pressure (PEEP) level.

During Proportional Pressure Support (PPS), a combination of two parameters, generate inspiratory pressure: flow assist (FA) and volume assist (VA).

Airway occlusion pressure (P 0.1) can be monitored during PPS and PAV+, but the work of breathing (WOB) cannot be monitored during PPS.

The transition from inspiration to expiration, or the cycling off criteria occurs when inspiratory flow decreases to a pre-set level between 1 to 10 liters per minute. Cycling of criteria in PAV+ should be adjusted around 10 liters per minute in obstructive patients, while around 1 liter per minute in restrictive and around 3–5 liters per minute in those without respiratory abnormalities.

If apnea occurs, the apnea ventilation is automatically activated as in other spontaneous modes.

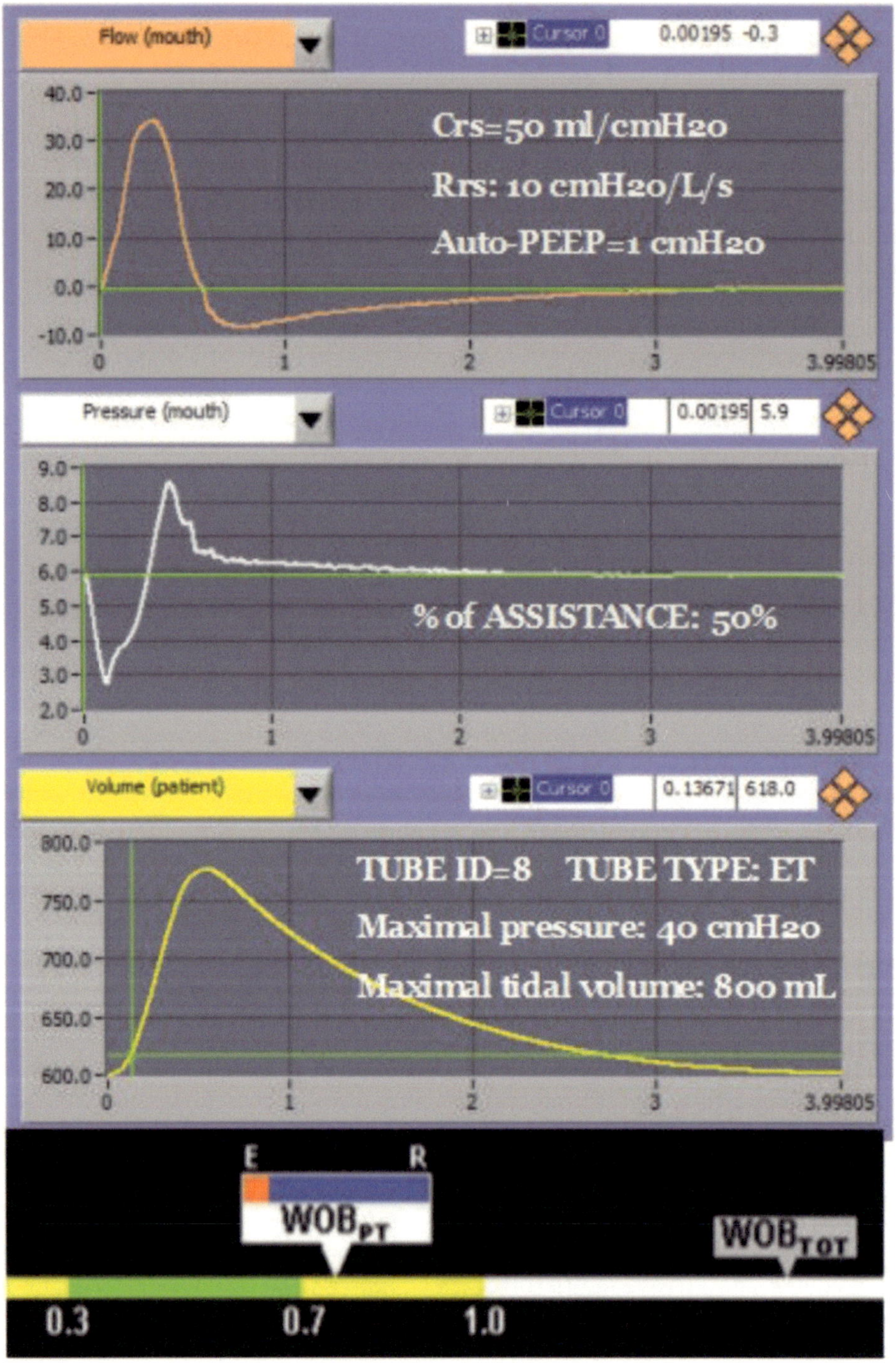

Figure 2.
PAV+ adjustments in clinical practice: parameters to set: % of assistance, tube ID, tube type, maximal pressure, maximal spontaneous tidal volume. Monitored parameters: compliance, resistance, auto-PEEP, work of breathing (J/liters). (Obtained from a simulator of the authors laboratory).

3.2 How to adjust parameters in PAV

In PAV+, the percentage support can be adjusted between 5 to 95%, usually between 10 and 20 to 70–80%. When percentage support is 50%, ventilator amplifies Pmus by two times, while when in 90%, Pmus is amplified by ten times. When the percentage support is set, patient and ventilator are sharing WOB, as defined by the operator. If the percentage support is 60%, the patient will be responsible by 40% of total WOB. The percentage support can be adjusted according to WOB, that can be kept between 0.3 to 0.7 joules/liter. However, WOB is considered normal between 0.2 to 1.0 J/L [10], and eventually, if others criteria are normal, like respiratory rate and P 0.1, percentage support not necessarily should be changed in case of WOB between 0.7 to 1.0 J/L (**Figure 2**). As the patient improves the percentage support is decreased to 20–30%; if the tidal volume remains 5–6 ml/kg/predicted body weight, respiratory rate less than 28, FIO2 less than 40%, PEEP less than 10 cmH20 and WOB less than 1.0 J/L, the patient can be extubated.

During Proportional Pressure Support (PPS), initially, the flow assistance (FA) should be set around 80% of airway resistance and volume assistance (VA), around 80% of elastance of the respiratory system, and then, changed according to the respective variations in these criteria. As higher FA and VA values, highest will be airway pressure and probably, tidal volume. PEEP and fraction of inspired oxygen (FiO2) should preferably be set in less than or equal to 10 cmH2O and 50% respectively.

3.3 Limitations, advantages and current evidences of PAV

PAV can also be used during noninvasive ventilation (NIV). As PAV requires clinical estimation of resistance and elastance, and measurements of these criteria with short end-inspiratory occlusions cannot be accurately performed in presence of leaks, it can, however, be of limited reliability [5]. Therefore, PAV as NIV did not present any evidence for daily routine.

Synchronism, proportional assistance and WOB monitoring seem to be the main advantages of PAV as well as to improve the patient-ventilator synchrony. Several studies and reviews evaluated PAV in comparison to PSV [7, 11–14] showing results favorable to PAV regarding synchronism, weaning success, sleep quality, duration of mechanical ventilation, lung and diaphragm protection and lower proportion of patients requiring reintubation [7, 11–14]. Although mortality seems to be generally favorable with PAV [11], this hypothesis has not been confirmed and more studies are necessary for this issue. One systematic review and meta-analysis that evaluated 14 randomized controlled studies, involving 931 patients [15] showed no difference on intubation risk (as noninvasive PAV), weaning time, hospital mortality, reintubation, or tracheostomy.

4. Neurally adjusted ventilatory assist (NAVA)

Neurally adjusted ventilatory assist (NAVA) is a mode of mechanical ventilation delivering pressure in response to the patient's respiratory drive, measured by the electrical activity of the diaphragm (EAdi) [16–18]. Initially described in 1999, by Christer Sinderby et al. [16], NAVA introduced a new dimension to mechanical ventilation, in which the patient's respiratory center can assume full control of the magnitude and timing of the mechanical support provided, regardless of changes in respiratory drive. This technology helps to decrease the risk of hyperinflation, respiratory alkalosis and hemodynamic impairment [16].

NAVA captures the EAdi, and uses it to assist the patient's breathing in synchrony with, and in proportion to respiratory drive [17–19]. Normal EAdi generally ranges between a few and 10 μV, while patients with chronic respiratory insufficiency may demonstrate signals 5–7 times stronger [17]. Although there is no cutoff for weaning outcome, EAdi above 26 μV can be related to failure [20].

Like PAV, there are no target tidal volume, mandatory rate and airway pressure preset. Ventilator support is proportional to a combination of EAdi, and NAVA level, which defines the magnitude of pressure delivered for a given EAdi [18]. NAVA depends of the captured signal of EAdi via sensing electrodes on a nasogastric tube [17] so, in case of damage on phrenic nerve or alterations on its activity, NAVA cannot be used.

Therefore, NAVA, like PAV, is also designated for patients with stable respiratory drive, and can be used in patients who are ventilated on PSV (as long as EADi is detected), or during weaning from mechanical ventilation. NAVA is also designated to improve synchronism, while generating proportional assistance to EAdi.

4.1 How NAVA works

A specialized nasogastric feeding catheter with electrodes should be inserted until the electrical activity of the crural diaphragm is observed [17, 21]. Correct positioning of the catheter is checked using the transesophageal electrocardiographies signal recorded by the electrodes as a guide [4], observed on the screen of the ventilator at second and third tracings. The absence of detectable EAdi is a contraindication of NAVA [17].

Ventilator support begins when EAdi starts [18]. As EAdi increases, assistance increases proportionally, and pressure delivered is cycled-off when EAdi is ended by the respiratory center (**Figure 3**) [17]. Application of a respiratory load, agitation, pain, respiratory distress or other causes that increase respiratory drive, can result in an increased EAdi, while over assistance should reduce EAdi [17].

NAVA trigger is not pneumatic as other ventilatory modes, but utilizes EAdi, a reflection of neural respiratory output to the diaphragm, as its primary source to trigger [17]. Pneumatic trigger is available, but electrical trigger of NAVA allows faster response to inspiratory effort than traditional pneumatic trigger.

When NAVA level is changed, the resulting pressure depends on how respiratory afferents modulate neural output to diaphragm [18]. If the response to an increase in NAVA level is not a reduction in EAdi, delivered pressure increases [17, 18]. In the presence of high inspiratory efforts (inspiratory pressures higher than 7 cmH20), when EAdi is at its highest, pressure delivered could reach extreme levels and may cause lung injury [18]. In this situation, NAVA and other spontaneous modes should be avoided.

Inspiratory pressure above PEEP level is adjusted automatically multiplying the EAdi by a proportionality factor, called NAVA level, expressed as cmH2O/μV [17, 22].

$$\text{Inspiratory pressure (above PEEP)} = \text{EAdi x NAVA level} \tag{2}$$

$$\text{Peak pressure} = \text{EAdi x NAVA level} + \text{PEEP} \tag{3}$$

For example: a NAVA level of 1 cmH2O/ μV will give an inspiratory pressure (above PEEP level) of 7 cmH2O when EAdi is 7 μV. Increasing NAVA level to 2 cmH2O/μV with the same EAdi will give an inspiratory pressure of 14 cmH2O.

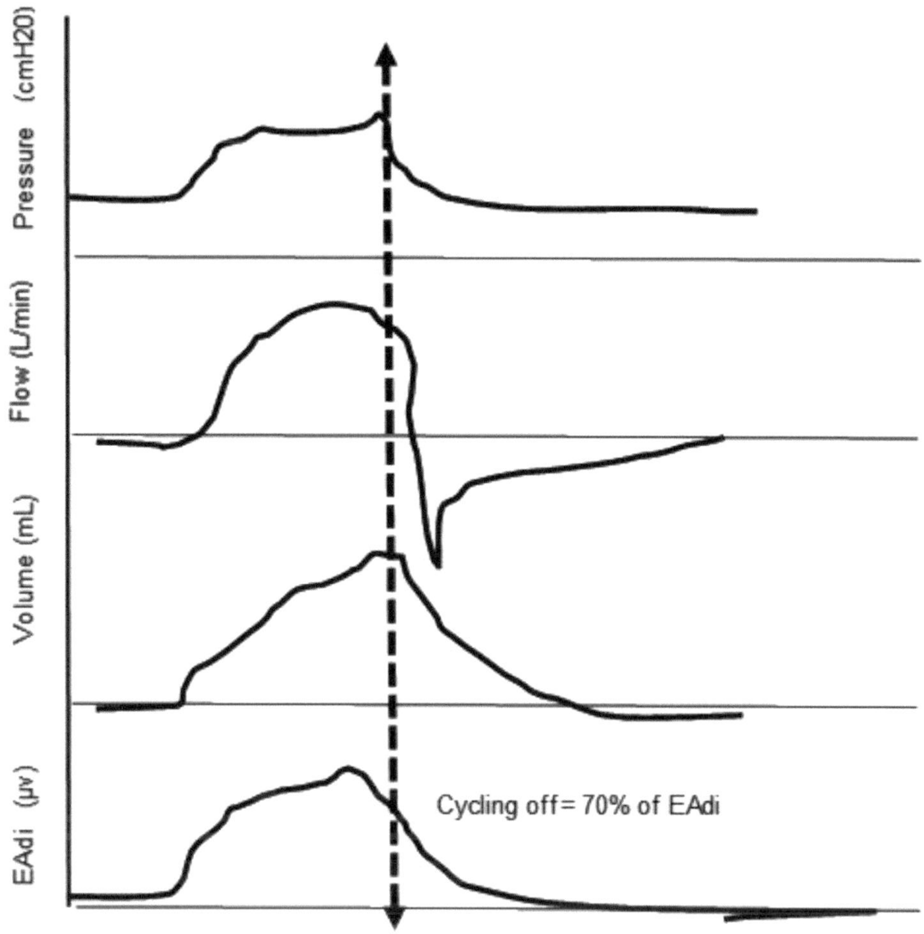

Figure 3.
NAVA curves in the clinical practice: pressure, flow, volume & EAdi (drawn by the author Carmen Barbas).

The transition from inspiration to expiration, or the cycling off criteria occurs when EAdi decreases automatically to 70–40% of the peak inspiratory flow value observed at the same breath, and cannot be modified by the operator [4, 17]. If apnea occurs, the apnea ventilation is automatically activated as in other spontaneous modes.

4.2 How to adjust parameters in NAVA

During NAVA, minimal and maximum EAdi are monitored constantly. The NAVA trigger detects increases in EAdi and should be set to a level where random variation in the background noise does exceed the trigger level. The neural inspiratory trigger default of 0.5 μV, or 0.5 μV above the minimal EAdi is adequate in most cases [4]. Auto-triggering is possible due to a too sensitive trigger setting and /or leak. In case of auto-triggering, neural inspiratory trigger can be slightly increased, until this asynchrony disappears.

Frequently, NAVA level is used between 0.5 to 2.0 μV/cmH2O [4, 19]. Initial value can be around 1.0 μV/cmH2O in most cases. There is no consensus as to best approach and no definitive recommendations are available how to set NAVA level." [4, 22]. Even so, some proposals deserve to be highlighted:

1. Pressure support that obtains 6 to 8 ml/kg predicted body weight during PSV, on ventilator function "NAVA preview" estimates the NAVA level that would achieve the same peak inspiratory pressure [4, 22].

2. To use NAVA level that generates 60 to 75% of maximal EAdi, observed during minimal inspiratory pressure of 3 to 7 cmH2O [22].

3. To use the minimal NAVA level associated with the absence of respiratory distress [4].

When inspiratory pressure reaches around 5 cmH2O, either by decreasing EAdi or decreasing NAVA level, weaning should be considered. PEEP and fraction of inspired oxygen (FiO2) should preferably be set in less than or equal to 10 cmH2O and 50% respectively.

4.3 Limitations, advantages and current evidence of NAVA

A limitation of NAVA mode is that it requires a specialized nasogastric feeding catheter with electrodes located in the esophagus for its functioning which adds additional costs. The advantages of NAVA mode are that it can monitor the EAdi (eletroactivity of diaphragm), it improves the inspiratory and expiratory synchrony and it can be used as a non-invasive ventilation (NIV) mode too [17]. Since EAdi is a pneumatically independent signal and not affected by leaks, NAVA can deliver assist synchrony during NIV even with leaks [17]. Only a few larger studies [23, 24] compare NIV-NAVA with NIV-PS. No improved clinical outcomes were observed except a decreased incidence of asynchronies in NIV-NAVA.

In a large, multicenter, randomized, controlled clinical trial that included patients with acute respiratory failure (ARF) from several etiologies [19], NAVA was used in 153 patients, while another 153 enrolled in the control group used volume control ventilation, pressure control ventilation, PSV, or pressure-regulated volume control. NAVA decreased duration of mechanical ventilation, although it did not improve survival in ventilated patients with ARF.

5. Adaptative support ventilation (ASV)

Adaptative Support ventilation (ASV) is a closed- loop controlled ventilatory mode, which is designed to ensure optimization of the patient work of breathing, automatically adjusted according to the patient's requirements. ASV combines passive ventilation with pressure-controlled ventilation with adaptive pressure support if the patient's respiratory effort is present.

ASV delivers pressure- controlled breaths according to the set minute ventilation, resulting in the best combination of tidal volume and respiratory rate. As the patient's inspiratory efforts start, ASV delivers pressure-supported breaths according to the set minute ventilation resulting in the best combination of tidal volume, respiratory rate and the patient's inspiratory effort. In ASV mode FIO2 and PEEP are set manually [25].

6. Intellivent-ASV

Intellivent ASV is also a closed-loop ventilation that adds the monitoring of SpO2 and Pressure End-tidal CO2 to best manage ventilation and oxygenation.

In Intellivent ASV mode the clinician sets patients' sex, height and choice the following respiratory mechanics situations: normal, ARDS, chronic hypercapnia and brain injury. Intellivent ASV determines the target PETCO2 and SPO2 according to the patient's condition. The ventilator controller adjusts the best tidal volume and respiratory rate to achieve the minute ventilation and PETCO2 set by the clinician combining pressure-control and or pressure support ventilation according to the patient's inspiratory effort. In Intellivent ASV, FIO2 and PEEP are adjusted according to the patient's SpO2 following a PEEP-FIO2 table [25].

7. Smart-care ventilation

Smart Care ® is an automatic weaning protocol, designed to stabilize the patient's spontaneous breathing in a comfort zone of a preset defined ventilation and to automatically reduce the ventilatory support. Smart Care ® ventilates the patient with pressure support which levels are adjusted according to respiratory rate, tidal volume and End tidal CO2 to meet the patient's demand. Smart Care ® classifies the patient a minimum of every 5 minutes into one of 8 categories and decreases or increases the pressure support levels accordingly. Smart Care® assesses and indicates the readiness for extubation after a successful automatic spontaneous breathing trial [26].

8. Conclusions

1. Volume assured pressure support ventilation can guarantee tidal volume with the advantages of pressure support variable inspiratory flow.

2. PAV+ can monitor the patient's respiratory compliance, respiratory resistance, auto-PEEP and work of breathing decreasing patient-ventilator asynchrony in comparison to PSV and other ventilatory modes. PAV plus allow lung and diaphragm protection, avoiding under and over-assistance.

3. NAVA allows the measurement of the patient's diaphragmatic eletroactivity and NAVA mode decreases patient-ventilator inspiratory and expiratory asynchrony.

4. ASV adjust pressure support, according to the respiratory rate to maintain the pre-set minute ventilation.

5. Intellivent-ASV adds the monitoring of PTCO2 and SpO2 and adjusts of pressure support according to respiratory rate to mantain the minute ventilation according to lung pathology.

6. Smart-care ventilation can automatically wean the patients, according to distinct patients classifications of lung pathology and indicates readiness for extubation.

Author details

Carmen Silvia Valente Barbas[1*] and Sergio Nogueira Nemer[2]

1 Pneumology and Critical Care, Albert Einstein Hospital, INCOR-University of São Paulo Medical School, São Paulo, Brazil

2 Pneumology, INCOR-University of São Paulo Medical School, São Paulo, Brazil

*Address all correspondence to: carmen.barbas@gmail.com

References

[1] Amato MB, Barbas CS, Bonassa J, Saldiva PH, Zin WA, de Carvalho CR. Volume-assured pressure support ventilation (VAPSV). A new approach for reducing muscle workload during acute respiratory failure. Chest. 1992 Oct; 102 (4): 1225-1234. doi: 10.1378/chest.102.4.1225.

[2] Younes M. Proportional assist ventilation: a new approach to ventilatory support: Theory. Am Rev Respir Dis 1992;145:114-120

[3] Ou-Yang LJ, Chen PO, Jhou HJ, Su VY, Lee CH. Proportional assist ventilation versus pressure support ventilation for weaning from mechanical ventilation in adults: a meta-analysis and trial sequential analysis. Crit Care 2020;24:256

[4] Rauseo M and Piquilloud L. Proportional modes. In: Heunks L and Schultz M. Handbook Invasive mechanical ventilation. The European Respiratory Society, First Edition 2019:62-73

[5] Schmidt M, Kindler F, Cecchini J, Poitou T, Morawiec E, Persichini R et al. Neurally adjusted ventilatory assist and proportional assist ventilation both improve patient-ventilator interaction. Crit Care 2015;19:56

[6] Younes M. Proportional Assist Ventilation. In: Tobin MJ. Principles and practice of mechanical ventilation. Mc Graw Hill. Second edition 2006: Chapter 13-335-364

[7] Vaporidi K. NAVA and PAV+ for lung and diaphragm protection. Curr Opin Crit Care 2019,25:000-000

[8] Kumar B, Vijayaraghavan T, Hamed S, Jain A, Chimunda T, Telias I, Friedrich JO, Burns KEA. Evidence supporting clinical use of proportional assist ventilation: a systematic review and meta-analysis of clinical trials. Journal of Intensive Care Medicine 2018:1-9

[9] Georgopoulos D, Xirouchaki N, Tzanakis N, Younes M. Data on respiratory variables in critically ill patients with acute respiratory failure placed on proportional assist ventilation with load adjustable gain factors (PAV+). Data on Brief 2016;8:484-493

[10] Brochard L, Martin GS, Blanch L, Pelosi P, Belda J, Jubran A et al. Clinical review: respiratory monitoring in the ICU – a consensus of 16. Crit care 2012,16:219

[11] Ou-Yang LJ, Chen PH, Jhou HJ, Su VYF, Lee CH. Proportional assist ventilation versus pressure support ventilation for weaning from mechanical ventilation in adults: a meta-analysis and trial sequential analysis. Crit Care 2020:24:556

[12] Pantazopoulos I, Mavrovounis G, Mermiri M, Kampolis C. Proportional assist ventilation versus pressure support ventilation for weaning from mechanical ventilation in adults: weaning success and mortality. Crit Care 2021:25:200

[13] Kataoka J, Kuriyama A, Norisue Y, Fujitani S. Proportional modes versus pressure support ventilation: a systematic review. Ann Intensive Care 2018:8:123

[14] Jonkman AH, Rauseo M, Carteaux G, Telias I, Sklar MC, Heunks M et al. Proportional modes of ventilation: technology to assist physiology. Intensive Care Med 2020. https://doi.org/10.1007/s00134-020-06206-z

[15] Kumar B, Vijayaraghavan T, Hamed S, Jain A, Chimunda T, T, Elias I et al. Evidence supporting clinical use of proportional assist ventilation:

a systematic review and meta-analysis of clinical trials. J Intensive care Med 2018:1-9

[16] Sinderby C, Navalesi P, Beck J, Skrobik Y, Comtois N, Friberg S et al. Neural control of mechanical ventilation in respiratory failure. Nature Medicine 1999; 5:1433-1436

[17] Sinderby C, Beck J. Neurally adjusted ventilatory assist (NAVA): an update and summary of experiences. Neth Crit Care 2007;11:243-252

[18] Sinderby C, Beck J, Spahija J, Marchie M, Lacroix J, Navalesi P et al. Inspiratory muscle unloading by neurally adjusted ventilatory assist during maximal inspiratory efforts in healthy subjects. Chest 2007;131:711-717

[19] Kacmarek RM, Villar J, Parrilas D, Alba F, Solano R, Liu S et al. Neurally adjusted ventilatory assist in respiratory failure: a randomized controlled trial. Intensive Care Med 2020: https://doi.org/10.1007/s00134-020-06181-5

[20] Barwing J, Pedroni C, Olgemoller U, Quintel M, Moerer O. Eletrical activity of diaphragm (EAdi) as a monitoring parameter in difficult weaning from respirator: a pilot study. Critical Care 2013,17:R182

[21] Hadfield D, Rose L, Reid F, Cornelius V, Hart N, Finney C et al. Factors affecting the use of neurally adjusted ventilatory assist in the adult critical care unit: a clinician survey. BMJ Open Resp Res 2020;07:e000783: DOI: 10.1136/bmjresp-2020-000783

[22] Terzi N, Piquilloud L, Rozé H, Mercat A, Lofaso F, Delisle S et al. Clinical review: update on neurally adjusted ventilatory assist – report of a round-table conference. Crit Care 2012;16:225

[23] Hansen KK, Jensen HI, Andersen TS, Christiansen CF. Intubation rate, duration of noninvasive ventilation and mortality after noninvasive neurally adjusted ventilatory assist (NIV-NAVA). Acta Anaesthesiol Scan 2020;64:309-318

[24] Prasad KT, Gandra RR, Dhooria S, Muthu V, Aggarwal AN, Aggarwal R et al. Comparing noninvasive ventilation delivered using neurally-adjusted ventilatory assist or pressure support in acute respiratory failure. Respir Care 2021;66:213-220.

[25] Arnal, JM, Kirakli C. Automed modes. In ERS Practical Handbook Invasive Mechanical Ventilation, 2019, pg.74-80

[26] Taniguchi C, Victor ES, Pieri T, Henn R, Santana C, Giovanetti E, Saghabi C, Timenetsky K, Caserta Eid R, Silva E, Matos GF, Schettino GP, Barbas CS. Smart Care™ versus respiratory physiotherapy-driven manual weaning for critically ill adult patients: a randomized controlled trial. Crit Care. 2015 Jun 11;19(1):246. doi: 10.1186/s13054-015-0978-6.

Section 2

Mechanical Ventilation in Specific Populations

Chapter 3

Mechanical Ventilation in the Trauma Patient

Jessica Lovich-Sapola, Jonathan A. Alter and Maureen Harders

Abstract

In this chapter, we discuss the unique ventilatory strategies of the trauma patient. Injuries can be direct to the lung resulting from the trauma or indirect because of other injury to the body. We will discuss the airway and ventilation management and concerns in a patient with chest trauma, abdominal trauma, head trauma, orthopedic, and burn injury. The chapter will explain lung-protective strategies as well as innovative ventilation management techniques including extracorporeal membrane oxygenation.

Keywords: trauma, ventilation, burn, anesthesia, chest

1. Introduction

Trauma lung injury can result from a direct injury to the lung or secondary to injury elsewhere. The trauma and the associated aggressive resuscitation lead to bleeding, edema, and inflammation of the lungs. The trauma can result in acute lung injury (ALI) and acute respiratory distress syndrome (ARDS). The goal of the ventilation is to preserve the lung as well as the brain and other organs that are injured. Each form of traumatic injury results in an individualized approach to mechanical ventilation [1].

1.1 Lung-protective ventilation strategies in the trauma patient

The primary goal of the trauma patient is to avoid hypoxia and secondary tissue injury. Mechanical ventilation may be initiated for reasons other than respiratory compromise, such as brain injury, shock, intoxication, agitation, or combativeness. Lung-protective ventilation strategies aim to reduce the volume and pressure delivered to the lung. For example, the goal tidal volume is 6–8 mL/kg of predicted body weight regardless of the type of ventilation [1].

1.2 Modes of ventilation in the trauma patient

Volume-controlled ventilation (VCV) is the most used form of ventilation in the operating room. The tidal volume (Vt), respiratory rate, and FiO_2 are set by the operator. This mode guarantees delivery of a set Vt and minute ventilation. The Vt is not reached if the peak inspiratory pressure (PIP) exceeds a set limit [1].

Pressure-controlled ventilation (PCV) can be used. In this type of ventilation, the Vt delivered is variable and depends on the airway resistance and the lung/chest wall compliance. This mode is recommended in the case of severe ARDS to promote better gas exchange [1].

Airway pressure release ventilation (APRV) is useful for the patient that has suffered a blunt trauma, with pulmonary contusions and severe atelectasis. APRV is also indicated for patients with morbid obesity and pregnancy. This mode of ventilation is a time-triggered, pressure-limited, and time-cycled mode of ventilation. The patient is able to breathe spontaneously. This mode is excellent for recruitment of the collapsed lung [1].

High-frequency oscillation ventilation (HFOV) results in the rapid delivery of very small tidal volumes with the application of high mean airway pressures. This type of ventilation results in active exhalation and therefore reduces air trapping. This type of ventilation is useful for patients with severe pulmonary contusion, ALI/ARDS, and smoke inhalation injury [1].

Noninvasive positive-pressure ventilation (NIPPV) including continuous positive airway pressure (CPAP) and bi-level airway pressure (BiPAP) can be used to treat acute respiratory failure. This mode of ventilation can be used in the trauma patient as well. This is not recommended for patients with brain injury, intoxication, or facial trauma. It is also not recommended for patients that are at increased risk of aspiration [1].

2. Chest trauma

Chest trauma, and the subsequent complications of chest injury, is significantly prevalent and the second most common cause of mortality in trauma. Injury sustained to the thorax can cause enormous damage to the heart, lungs, and major vasculature.

Any mechanism of injury to the chest wall or underlying organ systems has the potential to cause acute life-threatening issues with respiration. Mechanical ventilation, as it relates to the resulting complications of contusions, hypoxemia, and hemorrhage that occupy the spaces left behind by traumatic events, will be discussed throughout this chapter. Understanding the pernicious effects on respiratory mechanics and respiratory physiology helps the clinician to determine the timing of intubation and where the patient would most benefit on the spectrum of invasive ventilation.

2.1 Respiratory physiology in chest trauma

Injuries to the chest requiring mechanical ventilation may affect respirations in a variety of ways. Damage to the integument, musculoskeletal, nervous, or circulatory supply confined within and around the thoracic cavity can vastly change the physiology of respirations. Similarly, damage to the airways and lungs can significantly impede proper ventilation and oxygenation. As such, we can reduce respiratory compromise into two distinct circumstances: respirations compromised by altered mechanics of breathing, and respirations compromised by direct damage to the airway and lungs. Injuries to the respiratory system can also be categorized as being either penetrating or blunt in origin; however, the need for mechanical ventilation may exceed this distinction.

Integument provides a barrier from foreign organisms and elasticity, which is essential for expansion and contraction of the lungs; hindrance of integument by injuries, such as in the case of burns or circumferential eschars, limits the compliance of the respiratory system and often necessitates positive pressure ventilation.

Skeletal trauma most commonly involves rib fractures. Splinting, caused by painful respirations and often associated with factures involving the ribs, sternum, vertebrae, clavicles, or scapulae as well as injuries to soft tissue or muscle, can lead to atelectasis, hypoxemia, and pneumonia. Disruption to breathing mechanics by a flail chest, when two or more ribs are fractured in two or more places, and by hemo-pneumothorax, whereby the thoracic cavity is occupied by blood or air, may impede lung expansion and limit tidal volumes as well as oxygenation. Massive thoracic trauma is often accompanied by significant abdominal trauma. Diaphragmatic injury inhibits the lungs' ability to expand and contract. Invasion of the lung cavity by penetrating wounds, bone spurs, and the like creates a discordance within the respiratory system, inhibiting lung expansion, and reversing physiology to an open cavity [2].

Damage to respiratory parenchyma, including alveoli, alveolar ducts, and bronchioles, will impede gas exchange. High kinetic energy to the chest wall commonly causes pulmonary contusions and is the most frequently diagnosed intrathoracic injury associated with blunt trauma.

Tracheobronchial wounds, and more rarely esophageal damage, can have profound consequences. Structural damage may result in tension pneumothorax, pneumomediastinum, and subcutaneous emphysema. Most importantly, damage to the tracheobronchial tree can create an immediate threat to oxygenation and perfusion, a situation requiring swift discovery, appropriate intubation technique in a patient with diminished respiratory reserve, and isolation of injury for surgical manipulation, exposure, and repair.

Vascular injury, cardiac injury, and cardiac tamponade may impair circulation *via* massive hemorrhage, diminished preload because of decreases in venous return, and impediments to cardiac ejection from impedance on myocardium [3, 4].

2.2 Pulmonary contusion

Blunt trauma often results in pulmonary contusion. The early signs of tachypnea, rhonchi, wheezing, or hemoptysis may indicate pulmonary contusion. Changes may not be visible on a chest X-ray for up to 4–6 hours. Pulmonary contusions usually resolve in 7 days, which are managed easily by treating with permissive hypercapnia, conservative fluids, routine lung recruitment, positive end-expiratory pressure (PEEP), and lung-protective ventilation [1].

2.3 Hemothorax

The most common cause of a hemothorax is the rupture of intercostal vessels. Chest tube placement is recommended to access the rate of blood loss. Massive hemothorax, >1500 ml or one third of a patient's blood volume, often requires emergent surgery [1].

2.4 Bronchopleural fistulas

Bronchopulmonary fistula is a communication between proximal and distal airways and the pleural space. Mechanical ventilation can be difficult. The mean airway pressure should be kept low. Some experts recommend PCV due to the ability to control the pressure gradient more precisely. Lung isolation may be required if the leak is too large for proper ventilation. This can be achieved with main stem intubation, double-lumen tube, or bronchial blocker depending on the location of the fistula. The use of HFOV has been reported in some cases in addition to extracorporeal membrane oxygenation (ECMO) [1].

2.5 Choosing the appropriate mechanical ventilation for a chest trauma patient

2.5.1 Non-invasive ventilation

Provided the patient is hemodynamically stable without significant associated injury such as traumatic brain injury or severe abdominal trauma, non-invasive ventilation (NIV) techniques should be attempted. NIV has become common in acute chest trauma as it limits the hazard of further damaging the contused lung, which is at risk for diminished oxygenation and diffusion issues. Furthermore, NIV removes the risk of ventilator-induced lung injury, and many of the complications associated with endotracheal intubation should be considered prior to intubation attempts [5].

2.5.2 Indications for intubation

Respiratory compromise is depicted in many facets. Decreased tidal volume, increased respiratory rate, inadequate chest compliance, pleural compromise, failed lung mechanics, high oxygen requirements, and severe associated injuries (e.g., head trauma) are all situations that could require intubation. These indications are not absolute. These situations can quickly spiral out of ventilatory control. Surmounting a response prior to catastrophic failure and respiratory compromise is essential (**Table 1**) [6–8].

2.5.3 Ventilator settings in chest trauma

Initial ventilator settings in chest trauma are based on a lung-protective strategy. The Vt should be set between 4 and 8 mL/kg of ideal body weight with the plateau pressure < = 30 cm H_20. While positive end-expiratory pressure (PEEP) has well-established benefits in ICU and ARDS patients, it is initially withheld to evaluate the level of pulmonary injury, barotrauma, air leaks, and pulmonary shunt. The FiO_2 should be set = 1.0 and then titrated to an appropriate arterial oxygenation (PaO2). The respiratory rate should be set to 15–25 breaths per minute and then increased as need to achieve the desired PaCO2. Limiting plateau pressure to 30 cm H_20 will help protect lung physiology (**Table 2**) [6–8].

Indications for intubation in a chest trauma patient
• Hemodynamic instability
• Decreased respiratory reserves
• Hypoxemia (PaO_2 < 60 mmHg)
• Tachypnea
• Hypercarbia
• Glasgow coma scale of 8 or less

Table 1.
Indications for intubation in a chest trauma patient [6–8].

Initial ventilator settings in the chest trauma patient
• Tidal volumes between 4 and 8 mL/kg of ideal body weight
• $FiO_2 = 1.0$, titrated to arterial oxygenation
• Avoid PEEP
• Rate 15–25 breaths per minute

Table 2.
Initial ventilator settings in the chest trauma patient [6–8].

3. Abdominal trauma

Abdominal trauma can result from compression of the organs, deceleration injury, or penetrating trauma such as a stab or gunshot. It is important to first determine whether the injury is superior (above the diaphragm), inferior (inguinal ligament and symphysis pubis), or lateral (anterior axillary lines). The location of the injury helps to determine the organs involved [9].

The pain from an abdominal trauma can lead to poor shallow respirations, increased respiratory rate, and a decreased ability to clear secretions. This can result in a secondary pneumonia. The use of early mechanical ventilation has been correlated with a decreased risk of pneumonia, but after 5 days of ventilation that risk of pneumonia begins to increase again [10].

A patient presenting to the operating room with an abdominal injury requires a rapid sequence induction with intubation secondary to the high risk of aspiration. Most trauma patients are considered a "full stomach" and have delayed gastric emptying secondary to the high catecholamine levels from the stress of the trauma [9].

3.1 Abdominal compartment syndrome

Abdominal compartment syndrome can result from increased intra-abdominal pressure secondary to massive fluid resuscitation (bowel edema) or continued bleeding. Intra-abdominal pressures exceeding 20–25 mmHg can result in poor circulation and tissue perfusion as well as decreased cardiac output. The abdominal compartment syndrome can lead to respiratory dysfunction that will present as high peak pressures, decreased tidal volume, worsening atelectasis, and hypercarbia. Emergent surgery is required to release the abdominal pressure [9].

4. Head trauma

Traumatic brain injury (TBI) resulting from a trauma has a primary and secondary injury component. The primary injury results from the initial trauma and resulting mechanical deformation of the skull and brain tissue. The secondary injury is a result of the progressive insult to the neurons (**Table 3**) [11].

4.1 Brain injury and acute lung injury (ALI)

Head injury can occur as an isolated trauma or along with other injuries to the trauma patient. Isolated head injuries have been shown in clinical and experimental studies to cause lung damage soon after the injury. Neurogenic pulmonary edema can occur due to the release of catecholamines. In addition, the injured brain can display a systemic inflammatory response, which can result in injury to the

	Causes of brain injury
Primary brain injury	• Disruption of vascular structure • Compression of neuronal and glial tissue • Axonal injury
Secondary brain injury	• Astrocyte and neuronal swelling • Hypoperfusion • Increased free radicals • Inflammation • Cellular necrosis • Axonal degeneration • Systemic insults: hypotension, hypoxemia, hypoglycemia, hypocarbia, and hypercarbia

Table 3.
Causes of brain injury [11].

epithelial cells in the lungs. Subsequent mechanical ventilation (MV) can cause further pulmonary injury and strategies to minimize further damage to the lungs should be employed [12].

Mechanical ventilation in a patient with both a brain injury and ALI requires a balance between the principles that guide brain injury and the mechanical ventilation required to be protective of the lung. High PEEP can lead to elevated intrathoracic pressure, which results in decreased cerebral venous drainage and therefore poor cerebral perfusion. This effect is seen less in patients with ALI and ARDS; therefore, PEEP can often be safely applied in these patients. The key is to maintain the patient's volume status and mean arterial pressure. Also, the PEEP must be lower than the patient's intracranial pressure (ICP). The goal is to apply the lowest level of PEEP possible to still maintain oxygenation. Head elevation, avoiding tight endotracheal ties around the neck, and maintaining normocapnia are all important measures to monitor when ventilating a patient with head and lung injury [13].

Hypoxia, hypercarbia, and hypocarbia should be avoided in patients with a brain injury. Oxygenation should be monitored with a continuous pulse oximeter (goal >90%) and the PaO_2 should be >60 mmHg. Hyperventilation can result in cerebral vasoconstriction and brain ischemia. Prolonged hyperventilation is not recommended and should be avoided in the first 24 hours after injury. Hyperventilation should only be used as a temporizing measure [11].

4.2 Prolonged mechanical ventilation in the head injury patient

Prolonged mechanical ventilation in the patient with a traumatic brain injury presents a unique set of goals, first, to avoid further increased ICP and to optimize cerebral blood flow (CBF). Maintaining adequate oxygenation is critical to ensuring adequate cerebral perfusion pressure (CPP). Another goal is to reduce the risk of ARDS. In a multicenter study of ventilated patients with severe brain injury, higher tidal volumes were associated with increased risk of ALI. Lower PaO_2/FiO_2 ratio and higher respiratory rate were also independent predictors of ALI in the same study [14]. Low tidal volumes and permissive hypercapnia are recommended. One systemic review of intubated patients showed a tidal volume range of 6–8 ml/kg may reduce the risk of ARDS [15].

When ARDS develops along with TBI, management can be more difficult. ARDS NET strategies to improve ventilation can conflict with the goal of maintaining CPP.

Increasing PEEP up to 15 cm H_2O has a clinically insignificant effect on CPP; however, permissive hypoxia can lead to increased cerebral blood flow and increased CPP. ICP monitoring is suggested to monitor the effects of MV on CPP [12].

4.3 High-frequency percussive ventilation (HFPV) in head injury

Some studies show good results with HFPV in trauma patients with or without head injury. Using HFPV has resulted in improved oxygenation and reduced ICP [13].

5. Orthopedic trauma

Trauma management of a multiply-injured patient will require stabilization of pelvic and long bone fractures in as timely a manner that is safely possible. Research has shown that early stabilization of these fractures can reduce pain and improve patient outcomes. This includes a decrease in length of hospital stay and a reduction in pulmonary complications [16].

Patients with pre-existing pulmonary disease are at an even greater risk for significant pulmonary complications after a polytrauma. A chest X-ray or computed tomography (CT) scan is recommended on arrival to determine a baseline [16].

5.1 Fat embolism

Fat embolism syndrome (FES) is a result of the micro-embolism of fat and bone marrow from a patient's long bones [16]. Intraoperative transesophageal echocardiography performed on patients undergoing a long bone repair shows that most have some microembolization of fat and marrow [17]. This embolization can result in a varying degree of symptoms, including a significant acute inflammatory response [16, 17]. Most patients will not have a clinical impact. About 3–10% of patients will have clinically significant symptoms. The symptoms are usually progressive and develop over 12–72 hours. The most significant symptoms result in acute respiratory arrest and cardiac arrest [16].

The patient can present with hypoxia, tachycardia, mental status change, and a petechial rash. The rash is usually present on the upper body, including the conjunctiva, oral mucosa, neck, axilla, chest, and arms. Elevated pulmonary artery pressure and decreased cardiac output are seen with direct monitoring. When these symptoms arise, there are tests that can help confirm the diagnosis. These include testing for fat globules in the blood and urine, anemia, thrombocytopenia, and elevated ESR. A chest X-ray will often show bilateral alveolar infiltrates [16, 17].

The treatment for FES is supportive. The treatment for hypoxia requires early recognition and supplemental oxygenation, and may require ventilation management. Patients often require oxygen and PEEP. They may need long-term mechanical ventilation [16].

6. Burn injury

6.1 Smoke inhalational injury

Smoke inhalation is associated with increased mortality in a burn patient. Inhalational injury can be caused by the superheated air or the toxic compounds found in the smoke. These toxic compounds can include ammonia, sulfur, chlorine, and nitrogen dioxide [18].

There should be an increased suspicion of inhalational injury in any burn patient that presents with singed facial hair, carbonaceous deposits in the oropharynx, and blood carboxyhemoglobin levels greater than 10%. The chemical components of smoke can cause a significant inflammatory response that can lead to bronchospasm and impaired ciliary function. Lung necrosis and edema can lead to airway obstruction and atelectasis [19].

Signs and symptoms of inhalational injury include increased respiratory rate, increased secretions, stridor, dyspnea, use of accessory muscles, and facial burns. The first phase of inhalational injury includes asphyxia and acute toxicity. The second phase of inhalational injury begins at 24–96 hours after the injury and is the result of cellular level damage to the lungs. The treatment of inhalational injury includes ventilatory support, early pulmonary toilet, and nebulization therapy [18].

6.2 Carbon monoxide toxicity

Carbon monoxide is a byproduct of combustion. It is the cause of 80% of deaths associated with smoke inhalation from its ability to saturate hemoglobin at very low partial pressures. Burn patients with carbon monoxide toxicity may present with a normal pulse oximeter reading. It is important to always check arterial concentrations of oxy- and carboxy-hemoglobin. The treatment of carbon monoxide poisoning is oxygen therapy (**Table 4**) [18, 19].

6.3 Airway injury

Upper airway injury is often due to thermal heat injury. This leads to swelling and upper airway obstruction due to edema of the oropharynx (**Table 5**) [18].

Carbon monoxide saturation %	Symptoms
<15%	Rare symptoms
15–20%	Headache Nausea Confusion Tinnitus
20–40%	Neurological symptoms Disorientation Nausea Fatigue
40–60%	Cardiac dysrhythmias Brain injury Hallucinations Combativeness
>60%	Death

Table 4.
Carbon monoxide toxicity symptoms [18, 19].

Classic symptoms of impending airway obstruction:	• Stridor • Hoarseness • Dysphagia

Table 5.
Classic symptoms of impending airway obstruction in the burn patient [19].

Indications for immediate tracheal intubation:	• Respiratory distress and impending airway compromise (increased respiratory rate, increased secretions, stridor, dyspnea, and progressive hoarseness.) • TBSA burn >60% • Evidence of inhalational injury • Cardiovascular instability • Central nervous system depression

Table 6.
Indications for immediate tracheal intubation in the burn patient [18, 19].

6.4 Ventilator strategies in the burn patient

Patients with a large percentage of burn, burns to the head and neck, and inhalational injury will have an increased likelihood of need for mechanical ventilation. The large fluid load required to treat a burn can result in fluid overload to the lungs. Early bronchoscopy after intubation can help with the removal of secretions and burn-related debris and can help to reduce the length of time required for mechanical ventilation [10].

Non-invasive ventilation can be used for awake patients with minimal facial trauma that are stable hemodynamically. This can be started early upon arrival to the hospital (**Table 6**) [10].

Invasive mechanical ventilation can be lung-protective at low tidal volumes. Airway pressure release ventilation (APRV), high-frequency percussive ventilation (HFPV), and high-frequency oscillatory ventilation (HFOV) have been studied and shown useful in burn patients and to improve morbidity and mortality in comparison to VCV. These provide better oxygenation at lower FiO_2 than conventional ventilation with minimal effects on hemodynamics. APRV can be used to improve lung recruitment and oxygenation. There is no marked improvement in mortality, but it has been shown to stabilize alveoli, reduce edema of the alveoli, and helps to prevent the development of ARDS [10, 13].

6.5 Extubation of the burn patient

Extubation of a burn patient should be based on the patient hemodynamics, fluid resuscitation, inhalational lung injury, and existing airway abnormalities. Burn patients often receive large volumes of fluid resuscitation, which can result in airway edema. Burn patients also require large amounts of opioids for pain control. This results in burn patients often requiring prolonged intubation and ventilation. The criteria for extubation should be similar to those of non-burn patients: resolution of intoxications, ability to follow commands, pain-controlled, gag reflex, and appropriate cough. Burn patients need to be able to protect their airway from aspiration. An early tracheostomy should be considered for patients with long-term respiratory failure. While early tracheostomy has the benefits of improved communication, oral and tracheal hygiene, and improved patient comfort, it has not been associated with improved outcome [18, 19].

7. Extracorporeal membrane oxygenation (ECMO) in the trauma patient

Polytrauma is the leading cause of death among adults. This is often secondary to hemorrhagic shock, hypoxia, acute respiratory distress syndrome (ARDS), hypothermia, coagulopathy, and brain injury. The lung is often the first organ to fail in a severe trauma. ECMO has been used for nearly two decades, and its use has been gradually expanded to treat severe trauma patients, but the indications are uncertain and clinical outcomes are variable. The mortality of a severe trauma patient on ECMO is still high. There is much research needed on the proper initiation time for ECMO in the trauma patient and which patients will have the most benefit from ECMO. The safety and efficacy of ECMO still needs to be studied [20].

7.1 What is ECMO?

ECMO is a simplified version of the heart-lung machine used in open heart surgery. It is a method of gas exchange outside the body, so the lungs are exposed to minimal volume, pressure, rate, FiO_2, and they potentially have some time to recover [10]. ECMO can provide adequate tissue oxygenation, help in rewarming, and infuse large amounts of blood products quickly [20].

7.2 Complications of the trauma patient on ECMO

Complications associated with a trauma patient on ECMO include bleeding and thrombotic complications. Patients also presented with abdominal compartment syndrome, lung and brain edema, and pancreatitis [20].

8. Conclusion

As cases of severe trauma continue to increase, more and more trauma patients will be arriving in the operating rooms and intensive care units. It is important to understand how the mechanism of injury in a trauma affects the goals and types of mechanical ventilation required. The understanding of these individual cases will lead to improved patient outcomes.

Conflict of interest

The authors declare no conflict of interest.

Author details

Jessica Lovich-Sapola*, Jonathan A. Alter and Maureen Harders
MetroHealth Medical Center, Cleveland, Ohio, USA

*Address all correspondence to: jlsapola@gmail.com

References

[1] Dudaryk R, Weyers EW, McCunn M. Mechanical Ventilation of the patient following traumatic injury. In: Smith CE, editor. Trauma Anesthesia. 2nd ed. Cambridge: Cambridge University Press; 2015. pp. 340-351

[2] Brasel KJ, Moore EE, Albrecht RA, et al. Western trauma association critical decisions in trauma: Management if rib fractures. Journal of Trauma and Acute Care Surgery. 2017 Jan;**82**(1):200-203. DOI: 10.1097/TA.0000000000001301

[3] Edgecombe L, Sigmon DF, Galuska MA, et al. Thoracic trauma. In: StatPearls [Internet]. Treasure Island (FL): StatPearls Publishing. Last revision Jan 2021. Available from: https://www.ncbi.nlm.nih.gov/books/NBK534843/

[4] Weiser TG. Overview of thoracic trauma. In: Merck Manual Professional Version. [Internet]. Last full revision May 2020. Available from: https://www.merckmanuals.com/professional/injuries-poisoning/thoracic-trauma/overview-of-thoracic-trauma

[5] Chiumello D, Coppola S, Froio S, et al. Noninvasive ventilation in chest trauma: Systematic review and meta-analysis. Intensive Care Medicine. 2013;**70**:1171-1180. DOI: 10.1007/s00134-013-2901-4

[6] Richter T, Ragaller M. Ventilation in chest trauma. Journal of Emergencies, Trauma, and Shock. 2012;**4**(2):251-259. DOI: 10.4103/0974-2700.82215

[7] Prunet B, Bourenne J, David J-S, et al. Patters of invasive mechanical ventilation in patients with severe blunt chest trauma and lung contusion: A French multicentric evaluation of practices. Journal of Intensive Care Society. 2019;**20**(1):46-52. DOI: 10.1177/1751143718767060

[8] Rico FR, Cheng JD, Gestring ML, et al. Mechanical ventilation strategies in massive chest trauma. Critical Care Clinics. 2007;**23**:299-315

[9] Kaslow O. Anesthetic considerations for abdominal surgery. In: Varon A, Smith C, editors. Essentials of Trauma Anesthesia. 2nd ed. Cambridge: Cambridge University Press; 2018. pp. 232-245

[10] Arora S, Singh P, Trikha A. Ventilatory Strategies in Trauma Patients. Journal of Emergencies, Trauma, and Shock. 2014;**7**(10):25-31. DOI: 10.4103/0974-2700.125635

[11] Luk KHK, Dagal A. Anesthetic considerations for adult traumatic brian injury. In: Varon A, Smith C, editors. Essentials of Trauma Anesthesia. 2nd ed. Cambridge: Cambridge University Press; 2018. pp. 173-186

[12] Koutsoukou A, Katsiari M, Orfanos SE, et al. Respiratory mechanics in brain injury: A review. World Journal of Critical Care Medicine. 2016;**5**(1):65-73. DOI: 10.5492/wjccm.v5.i1.65

[13] Mohta M. What's new in emergencies, trauma, and shock? Mechanical ventilation in trauma patients: A tight-rope walk! Journal of Emergencies, Trauma, and Shock. 2014;**7**(1):1-2. DOI: 10.4103/0974-2700.125630

[14] Mascia L, Zavala E, Bosma K, et al. High tidal volume is associated with the development of acute lung injury after severe brain injury: an international observational study. Critical Care Medicine. 2007;**35**:1815-1820. DOI: 10.1097/01.ccm.0000275269.77467.df

[15] Fuller BM, Mohr NM, Drewry AM, et al. Lower tidal volume at initiation of

mechanical ventilation may reduce progression to acute respiratory distress syndrome: A systemic review. Critical Care. 2013;**17**(1):R11. DOI: 10.1186/cc11936

[16] Lovich-Sapola JA, Smith CE. Anesthesia for Orthopedic Trauma. In: Al-Aubaidi Z, editor. Orthopedic Surgery. Rijeka: InTech; 2012. pp. 185-220

[17] Lovich-Sapola JA, Smith CE. Anesthetic considerations for musculoskeletal trauma. In: Varon A, Smith C, editors. Essentials of Trauma Anesthesia. 2nd ed. Cambridge: Cambridge University Press; 2018. pp. 246-260

[18] Lovich-Sapola J. Anesthesia for burns. In: Smith CE, editor. Trauma Anesthesia. 2nd ed. Cambridge: Cambridge University Press; 2015. pp. 666-688

[19] Olivar H, Sharar S. Anesthetic management of the burn patient. In: Varon A, Smith C, editors. Essentials of Trauma Anesthesia. 2nd ed. Cambridge: Cambridge University Press; 2018. pp. 261-274

[20] Wang C, Zhang L, Qin T, et al. Extracorporeal membrane oxygenation in the trauma patients: A systematic review. Journal of Emergency Medicine. 2020;**15**:51. DOI: 10.1186/s13017-020-00331-2

Chapter 4

Ventilation Strategies in Obese Patients

Pavol Pobeha

Abstract

Obesity is an increasingly prevalent disease and is a root and complication of conditions necessitating mechanical ventilation. Obese patients require a careful approach due to the particular manner of how ventilatory mechanics is affected, if obstructive sleep apnea (OSA) is present. The two main diagnoses we may encounter while ventilating these patients are obesity hypoventilation syndrome (OHS) and chronic obstructive pulmonary disease (COPD) in an obese patient, which has been recently proposed as a novel phenotype of COPD. The excessive amount of fat in the abdomen, chest wall, and around upper airways warrants the use of special ventilation modes and settings. This chapter provides insight into which issues should be considered when ventilating an obese patient, either in acute or chronic conditions. We stress the importance of acknowledging the high risk of OSA and how OSA affects the ventilation algorithms.

Keywords: non-invasive ventilation, obesity hypoventilation syndrome, COPD, overlap syndrome, sleep-disordered breathing, ventilation strategies

1. Introduction

Obesity is a disease with prevalence increasing significantly; about a third of the world's population is overweight or obese. The number of obese people has doubled in the last 20–30 years, and this trend continues [1]. This is closely related to the increase in the number of obese patients admitted to the intensive care units (ICU) as well as those requiring mechanical ventilation. The specificity of obesity in critically ill patients lies in the increased risk of infections, impaired respiratory drive, respiratory mechanics as well as the presence of sleep-disordered breathing [2]. A frequently mentioned diagnosis linking respiratory failure and obesity is obesity hypoventilation syndrome (OHS), but obesity also affects patients with other diseases, including respiratory and lung diseases. It is necessary to mention patients with chronic obstructive pulmonary disease (COPD), where a subset of obese patients benefits from a different approach to diagnosis and treatment compared to low-weight patients. This chapter aims to clarify the issue of respiratory failure in obesity and its treatment using mechanical ventilation in both acute and chronic conditions.

2. Mechanisms of respiratory failure development in obesity

The development of respiratory failure in obesity is a gradual and often long-term process. Although the proportion of individual factors may vary from patient to patient, the disease results from a complex of the following mechanisms [3–6]:

- Reduction of vital capacity and functional residual capacity due to the mass of abdominal and subcutaneous chest fat
- Upper airway narrowing and collapse during sleep—obstructive sleep apnea (OSA)
- Accumulation of fat deposits in the respiratory system with increased lower airways resistance
- Increased work of breathing (increased respiratory load)
- Hypoxic pulmonary vasoconstriction
- Fluid overload associated with nocturnal rostral fluid shift
- Rapid eye movement (REM) associated hypoventilation
- Impaired respiratory mechanics—muscle weakness
- Central leptin resistance—deterioration of the respiratory drive
- Accumulation of serum bicarbonate—reduction of ventilatory response to carbon dioxide (CO_2)

All these pathomechanisms affect the development and course of the disease in individual patients and should be considered in the diagnosis and treatment of respiratory failure and the setting of ventilation strategies. Guideline for mechanical ventilation generally distinguishes recommendations for the treatment of patients with obstructive pulmonary disease and restrictive diseases and separately for the diagnosis of obesity hypoventilation syndrome [7–9]. However, as obesity is present in various diseases and the above-mentioned pathomechanisms contribute to the clinical picture, in the following, we will mention the specifics of the treatment of respiratory failure in multiple diseases.

3. Obesity hypoventilation syndrome

Obesity hypoventilation syndrome is standardly defined by the combination of:

- Obesity with body mass index (BMI) ≥ 30 kg m^{-2}.
- Daytime hypercapnia—arterial CO_2 tension ($PaCO_2$) ≥ 45 mm Hg.
- Sleep-disordered breathing.
- The diagnosis of OHS cannot be made if an alternative explanation for hypoventilation (e.g., neuromuscular, mechanical, or metabolic disease) is present [10].

As the development of hypoventilation in OHS is gradual, the diagnosis is in most cases made at a stable stage, when the patient is examined in a sleep laboratory for symptoms of sleep-disordered breathing [10]. Approximately one-third of patients are diagnosed at the point of acute-on-chronic hypercapnic respiratory failure [11], and these patients often require critical care. Comorbidities such as heart failure (usually with preserved ejection fraction), pneumonia, and sepsis contribute to the acute condition. A major problem in the acute and long-term management of these patients is that instead of making a correct diagnosis of OHS, other diseases such as COPD or asthma are misdiagnosed [12, 13]. The misdiagnosis of obstructive pulmonary disease without adequate lung function examination incorrectly directs treatment to the application of bronchodilators instead of adequate respiratory support.

3.1 Classification of OHS patients

Based on the presence of OSA and hypoventilation, three phenotypes of patients with OHS were observed [14, 15]:

- **Severe OSA**—free of REM sleep hypoventilation. This phenotype is characterized by a lack of CO_2 washout capacity after obstructive apnea episodes.

- **Isolated OHS**—characterized by morbid obesity (BMI often ≥40 kg m^{-2}), severe hypercapnia and REM sleep hypoventilation without the presence of OSA.

- **Combined OHS and OSA**.

Polysomnographic (PSG) findings for individual phenotypes are shown in **Figure 1**.

Figure 1 describes the excerpts of polygraphic recordings displaying from the top oxygen saturation, thoracic respiratory effort, airflow, and snoring. The first excerpt of severe OSA is exhibiting short interapneic intervals with oxygen saturation rising above 90%. The second excerpt illustrates low baseline oxygen saturation with further desaturations after apneic events. The third excerpt shows low baseline saturation with no desaturations reflecting isolated hypoventilation.

The classification is based on observations and medical evidence. It is a fact that a significant proportion of patients with OHS have concomitant OSA (near 70%

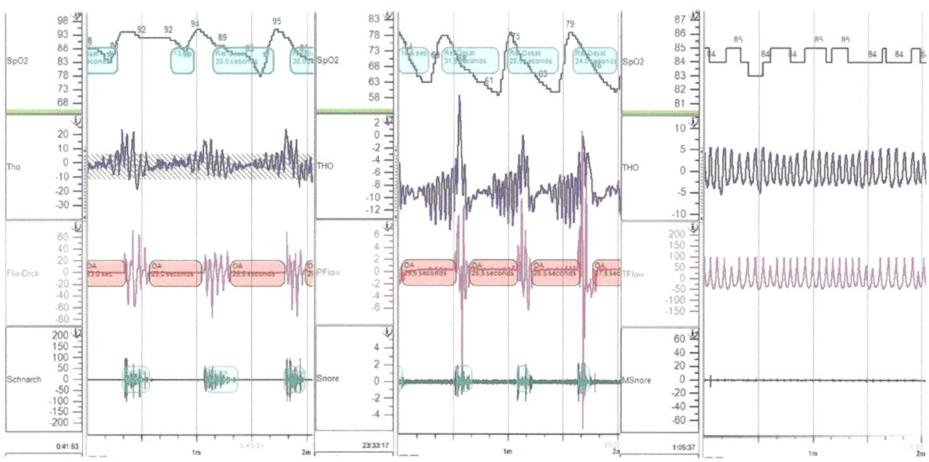

Severe OSA | Combined OSA and hypoventilation | Isolated hypoventilation

Figure 1.
Phenotypes of OHS.

of patients have severe OSA), and its presence should be presumed in treatment, especially in acute situations [14]. In a stable state, it is appropriate to devote time to the precise diagnosis, differential diagnosis, and titration of treatment.

3.2 Ventilation strategies in acute hypercapnic respiratory failure and OHS

While continuous positive airway pressure (CPAP) treatment may be appropriate for OHS and chronic hypercapnic respiratory failure, noninvasive ventilation (NIV) is the method of choice for acute or acute-on-chronic respiratory failure. It is a better alternative to invasive ventilation because it significantly reduces patient morbidity and mortality and reduces the risk of reintubation [7, 15].

3.2.1 Indications for NIV in acute hypercapnic respiratory failure in OHS

In an obese patient with a known or suspected diagnosis of OHS who meets the criteria for initiating ventilation support, noninvasive ventilation should be considered the first treatment modality.

Acute ventilatory support in OHS patients is indicated if the following criteria are met [16]:

- $PaCO_2 \geq 45$ mm Hg.
- Respiratory acidosis with $7.1 < pH < 7.35$.
- Severe breathlessness, tachypnea (≥23 breaths per min).

3.2.1.1 Notes

- Severe respiratory acidosis increases the risk of NIV failure but is not an obstacle to this treatment. It is possible to start a trial with NIV and be prepared for urgent endotracheal intubation.
- NIV can also be indicated in some hospitalized obese hypercapnic patients with daytime somnolence, sleep-disordered breathing, and/or right heart failure in the absence of respiratory acidosis [17].

3.2.2 Examinations and procedures before the start of the NIV

Before starting treatment with NIV, it is necessary (assuming patient safety—no delay of NIV) to perform the following procedures:

- Blood collection for arterial blood gas (ABG) analysis. An arterialized capillary blood sample (e.g., by heat) is an alternative
- Electrocardiography (12 lead)
- Chest radiography
- Search for and treatment of reversible causes of respiratory failure
- To determine in advance an individual plan for possible escalation of treatment (e.g., for do not intubate patients) [17]

3.2.3 Management of NIV in acute OHS patient

In the case of acute OHS, the NIV should be started immediately. OHS patients with severe daily sleepiness may be so somnolent that they cannot participate in placing their face masks. Treatment should be provided by staff experienced in NIV, and the patient should be placed in a high dependency unit (HDU) or intensive care unit (ICU) for close monitoring [17].

3.2.3.1 Important notes on the management of acute NIV in OHS

- **Interface**—Face mask (oronasal/full-face mask) is preferred in acute settings and very obese patients because of high pressures and mouth breathing [15]. Proper mask fitting is the key to successful NIV. It is advisable to choose the appropriate size mask (masks too large for the patient's face are more likely to leak) and adjust the restraining straps so that the mask is so loose that it seals well. In the case of skin lesions or bruises with an oronasal mask, it is possible to try the rotation of the masks (regular alternation of different masks; for example, total face mask or under nose full-face mask—e.g., Amara view, Dreamwear full-face—Philips Respironics™).

- **Ventilation mode**—Ventilation modes with backup respiratory rate are recommended in acute settings, for example, spontaneous-timed (ST) or pressure controlled (PC) mode, depending on the ventilation device and physician's experience.

- **Expiratory positive airway pressure (EPAP)/positive end-expiratory pressure (PEEP)**—It should be at least 8 cm H_2O [7, 15, 17]. It is possible to start with pressure 6 cm H_2O and gradually titrate upwards to improve tolerance and oxygenation, reduce respiratory load and control upper airway obstruction (snoring reduction). EPAP higher than 13–14 cm H_2O can be poorly tolerated, and too high EPAP reduces the possibility of achieving sufficient pressure support (depending on the ventilation device). Since comorbid sleep apnea is present in sleep, it is necessary to optimize EPAP during sleep. Software analysis of ventilation is helpful in subsequent parameter adjustments. Effective EPAP can be titrated manually, alternatively using specific modes, for example, AVAPS AE™ (Philips Respironics) or auto-ST (Löwenstein medical) [18].

- **Inspiratory positive airway pressure (IPAP)**—It should be initiated at least 8 cm H_2O higher than EPAP. The difference between EPAP and IPAP, that is, pressure support (PS), should be increased gradually (up to 30 cm H_2O) to achieve a sufficient chest wall excursion and tidal volume (measured or estimated by a ventilator), but patient tolerance must be achieved [11, 15, 16].

- **Ensuring the target volume**—The use of ventilation pressure-controlled modes with target tidal volume settings such as average volume assured pressure support-AVAPS™ (Philips Respironics) or target volume (Löwenstein medical) is not necessary. However, in extremely obese patients with marked respiratory asynchrony in NIV, these modes can be used, as the ventilator can compensate for changes in lung compliance (e.g., patient position changes or tidal volume variability in-breaths triggered spontaneously or by device). Target tidal volume should be calculated and targeted at 8 (maximum 10) mL kg^{-1} ideal body weight [15]. PS (IPAP settings—IPAP minimum-maximum) should be in an acceptable range (starting 4 cm H_2O above EPAP) to allow the device to reach the desired tidal volume. The rate of pressure change (to adjust tidal volume) is suitable to choose medium to fast. Volume-targeted ventilation modes are accompanied by higher mask air leaks but can (assuming good mask fitting) improve breathing synchronization instead of changing to other modes.

- **Backup rate**—Setting the backup respiratory rate in the range of 12–14 is the prevention of central apnea and hypoventilation during sleep [19].

- **Inspiratory time**—For mandatory breaths should be at least 1.2 s (up to 1.5 s). For ventilation devices with the possibility of setting the inspiratory and expiration ratio (I-E ratio), it is suitable to set it 1:2–1:1 [20].

- **Oxygen**—Oxygen inhalation is an extreme risk for OHS patients as it worsens hypoventilation [21]. In the stable and acute stage, oxygen is considered an additional treatment to NIV. In acute NIV, the amount of oxygen must be increased gradually to achieve saturation above 90% [11, 14–16].

- **Forced diuresis**—In acute-on-chronic respiratory failure in OHS, fluid overload commonly contributes to the severity of the disorder. Forced diuresis may be helpful initially [17].

- **Phlebotomy**—Hyperviscosity associated with secondary erythrocytosis may impair oxygen delivery in OHS patients. Phlebotomy may be considered in a patient with very high hematocrit as a part of intensive care therapy, provided that NIV is treated effectively and with sufficient oxygenation [11].

3.2.3.2 Contraindications to the use of NIV

Absolute:

- facial burns, severe facial deformity—inability to put on a mask
- gastrointestinal bleeding or ileus
- significant hemoptysis
- undrained pneumothorax
- inability to protect the airway, for example, fixed airway obstruction

Relative:

- copious respiratory secretions
- hemodynamic instability (cardiogenic shock, myocardial infarction)
- severe hypoxemia and acidosis ($pH < 7.1$)—predictors of NIV failure
- confusion/agitation
- coma—however, hypercapnic coma can be reversed using NIV [22, 23]

3.2.3.3 Monitoring in acute NIV

Patients treated with NIV require intensive care and careful monitoring, including:

- Monitoring: Respiratory rate, oxygen saturation, end-tidal CO_2, blood pressure, transcutaneous measurement of carbon dioxide ($TCCO_2$)

- Observation: Dyspnea, paradoxical abdominal movements, mask leaks, asynchrony with ventilator

- Measurements: Glasgow coma scale (GSC), acute physiology and chronic health evaluation (APACHE) score

- Labs: Blood gas analysis (sampling after 1–2 h of NIV, followed by 6–12 h for the first 24 h)

- Waveforms: Analysis of NIV parameters [23]

3.2.3.4 Failure of acute NIV and indication of endotracheal intubation in OHS

Despite careful monitoring and proper ventilation, NIV failure may occur in some cases. There is no exact algorithm to determine when to indicate intubation, but it is necessary to know the most common predictors of NIV failure [23–25]:

- excessive unintentional air leaks

- high severity score on admission (pH < 7.25, APACHE II score > 29)

- excessive respiratory secretions

- intolerance and noncompliance with NIV

- polymorbidity

- severe hypoxemia and low level of $PaCO_2$

- pneumonia

- low level of bicarbonates (HCO_3)—possible link to renal failure

- short duration of NIV

- minimal or no change in pH after 1–2 h of NIV

- no reduction in respiratory rate after 1–2 h of NIV

3.2.3.5 Further recommendations after successful acute ventilation in OHS

Data show that patients with a diagnosed or suspected diagnosis of OHS have a higher risk of death if they are discharged from the hospital without home positive airway pressure (PAP) treatment. Therefore, it is appropriate to set these patients for NIV treatment (ideally with pressure settings as in hospitalization or with auto-PAP settings) and to schedule an early examination in the sleep laboratory and titration of PAP treatment (within 3 months) [26]. In patients acutely ventilated invasively, the use of NIV is an appropriate weaning strategy, as it effectively prevents respiratory failure in the first 48 h after extubation [24]. In patients requiring tracheostomy for prolonged invasive ventilation, it is advisable to perform decannulation and adjustment to home NIV after successful weaning instead of indicating long-term mechanical ventilation via tracheostomy.

3.3 Ventilation strategies in chronic hypercapnic respiratory failure and OHS

Initiating treatment of OHS patients in a stable stage allows assessing the ventilation strategy carefully. The choice of appropriate treatment should be based upon the severity of clinical state, the laboratory, functional and polysomnographic findings, reasonable cost-effectiveness, and the physician's experience. Clinical practice and literature data do not favor treatment by either CPAP or NIV as they are comparable, though some studies acknowledge certain benefits of NIV over CPAP.

3.3.1 Comparison of effectivity of CPAP and NIV

In the medium-term treatment, both CPAP and NIV have improved:

- Daytime hypercapnia, sleepiness [27]
- Health-related quality of life [28]
- Polysomnographic measures [29]
- Structural and functional echocardiographic measures [30]

NIV was superior to CPAP in terms of:

- Lung functions and 6 min walking test
- The rapidity of blood gases improvement [28]

In the long-term treatment, both CPAP and NIV have improved:

- Number of hospitalization days [31]
- Pulmonary hypertension and left ventricular diastolic dysfunction [32]

The concerns about the potentially harmful effect of NIV of hemodynamics due to the application of unphysiological positive pressure have been addressed by utilizing impedance cardiography, but it has not shown any deleterious impact on ventricular function [33].

The one undeniable benefit of CPAP over NIV is its lower cost [34]. The novel guidelines for the management of OHS by the American Thoracic Society [26] propose a switch of treatment from NIV to CPAP once the patient has achieved significant clinical improvement. This switch has been shown to be feasible and even favored by patients [35].

3.3.2 Obstructive sleep apnea

The one defining feature of OHS is its high prevalence of OSA, mainly of severe degree (estimated in around 70% of OHS patients). Thus, in patients with an apnea-hypopnea index (AHI) cut-off ≥30 episodes/h, it is reasonable to start with CPAP, as the primary aim is to alleviate obstruction in the upper airways, which might lead to the eventual resolution of chronic hypercapnia. For the patients without severe OSA, we should aim to improve the mechanics in the respiratory system and depression of the respiratory center; that is why NIV is used as an initial treatment.

3.3.3 Failure of CPAP

The patients initially set on CPAP should be monitored for signs of CPAP failure. In that case, a switch to NIV is warranted. The definition of CPAP failure is inconsistent among different researchers. Some of the criteria used for CPAP failure in OHS patients were:

- Insufficient improvement of oxygen saturation on CPAP:
    - Oxygen saturation below 90% for more than 20% of total sleep despite adequate abolition of apneas and hypopneas [36]
    - Oxygen saturation < 85% or hypercapnia despite maximal CPAP [37]
    - Oxygen saturation below 90% for more than 30% of titration night [38]
    - Oxygen desaturation < 80% over 10 min [9]
- Persistence of apneic and hypopneic episodes [37]
- Insufficient improvement of CO_2 levels
    - ≥5 min-long increase in nocturnal $PTcCO_2 > 55$ mm Hg and in $PaCO_2 \geq 10$ mm Hg compared to the awake state [9]
    - Daytime $PaCO_2 > 45$ mm Hg [38]

The choice of criteria for CPAP failure should be suited for the practice of a particular sleep laboratory, and it should be consistent over time.

Careful evaluation is necessary to avoid deeming inadequate patient compliance as CPAP failure.

It is important to note that a failure of CPAP during titration does not necessarily lead to failure of the CPAP treatment [36]. A single or few titration nights of CPAP may falsely display a failure, when in fact, a more extended period of treatment (2–3 months) might be necessary for CPAP to be effective. The length of a trial should be adapted according to the convenience of a sleep laboratory.

3.3.3.1 Predictors of CPAP failure

The high proportion of CPAP failure in OHS patients has led to identifying certain predictors when CPAP should be tried with a reasonable expectation of success and when to proceed straight to NIV.

Recognized CPAP failure predictors were:

- awake oxygen saturation < 94% and $PaO_2 < 68$ mm Hg [37]
- daytime $PaCO_2 > 53$ mm Hg [15]
- BMI ≥ 50 kg m^{-2} [15, 39]
- significant comorbidities [40]
- acute respiratory failure [39]
- and clinician's preference [39]

Generally, worse blood gases [38], higher obesity, significant comorbidities, and clinician's preference warrant the trial of NIV in the first step.

3.3.4 Setup strategies of NIV

Novel increasingly intelligent auto-titrating devices are able to adjust to a patient's ventilatory need depending on his/her body position or the sleep stage.

- Volume targeted pressure support assures sufficient ventilation but may potentially lead to sleep disturbance.
- Auto-titrating EPAP allows to maintain the patency of upper airways and alleviates concomitant sleep apnea [18].
- Standard ST mode is not inferior to the novel modes but requires precise and gradual titration, which is time-consuming.

Similarly, as the OHS patients are monitored for signs of CPAP failure, patients with NIV should be checked frequently, as there is a possibility of improvement of the respiratory center sensitivity, and a switch from NIV to CPAP might be considered.

4. Chronic obstructive pulmonary disease (COPD)

COPD is a serious disease with an increasing prevalence, accompanied by a high risk of respiratory failure [41]. Unlike OHS, COPD is a disease where, in addition to the failure of the ventilatory pump (muscle weakness, shortening of the diaphragm), lung disease (obstructive airway disorder) is added [42]. The severity of the situation and the fact that it is a progressive disease also affect the management of respiratory failure. The use of NIV in COPD is common practice today. This treatment has clearly been shown to be effective in acute exacerbations of COPD (AECOPD) [43] and has long been a controversial topic in chronic indications [44]. However, recent studies have provided clear evidence in favor of treatment (including the effect on survival), and the greatest benefit of NIV has been present with higher pressures in NIV settings for maximum CO_2 reduction, in patients with higher basal $PaCO_2$ values, and in those who achieve high treatment compliance [45–47]. In the management of hypercapnic respiratory failure in COPD, there is growing evidence of the effectiveness of so-called high-intensity NIV (HI-NIV) [48].

However, many studies and guidelines perceive COPD as a single disease and do not reflect the existence of different phenotypes, comorbidities, and the need for a unique approach to them. One of them is an obese patient with COPD.

4.1 Obese patient with COPD

Several respiratory societies perceive COPD, not as a single homogeneous airway disease but also distinguishes between several phenotypes characterizing differences between patients [49, 50]. In intensive care units, patients with COPD often appear to be classified as a classic "Blue bloater." These patients are generally classified as chronic bronchitis phenotype, but its definition does not fully describe such a complex clinical trait. On the contrary, there is increasing evidence that this trait of COPD patients is characterized by different radiological findings than those seen in emphysema, and it is associated strongly with obesity and frequently also with OSA [51]. The prevalence of obesity among COPD patients is also very high and variable (18–54%) [51, 52]. Obesity is strongly linked with the presence of OSA, and in COPD patients requiring inpatient pulmonary rehabilitation, the number of obese patients with OSA increases significantly [53]. The presence of obesity and the COPD-OSA overlap syndrome appears to be a key factor in the pathogenesis and development of clinical signs of the blue bloater trait. This statement is underlined with evidence that the severity of static hyperinflation is negatively associated with the apnea-hypopnea index in both COPD and non-COPD patients surviving acute hypercapnic respiratory failure [54]. This evidence is following data showing that overlap syndrome increases the risk of respiratory failure, pulmonary hypertension, and COPD exacerbations [55]. In line with the above literary data [56], a new "obese patient with COPD" phenotype (characterized by predominantly chronic bronchitis, less hyperinflation, metabolic and cardiovascular comorbidity, sleep apnea symptoms, that is, daytime sleepiness, snoring, nonrefreshing sleep, and/or hypercapnic respiratory failure) was proposed [57] with a recommendation of screening for sleep-disordered breathing in this group of patients [50].

4.2 Ventilation strategies in acute exacerbation of COPD in obese patients

Acute exacerbation of COPD (AECOPD) is a severe condition that requires urgent intervention, and recommendations for its treatment are well known [41]. NIV has an irreplaceable place in the management of AECOPD in the event of acute or acute on chronic respiratory failure [17, 43]. In a patient with COPD who is obese, it should be borne in mind that obesity is probably one of the predominant factors predisposing to respiratory failure. Other possible factors such as cardiogenic edema, infection, uncontrolled excessive oxygen therapy, or pneumothorax should not be forgotten [17]. Because NIV effectively prevents endotracheal intubation and survival in patients with AECOPD [23, 58], it should be indicated whenever a patient meets the criteria for initiation.

4.2.1 Indications for NIV in acute hypercapnic respiratory failure in COPD

Acute ventilatory support in AECOPD is indicated in the same criteria as in OHS patients:

- $PaCO_2 \geq 45$ mm Hg
- Respiratory acidosis with $7.1 < pH < 7.35$
- Severe breathlessness, tachypnea (≥23 breaths/min)

4.2.1.1 Notes

It should be emphasized that controlled low-flow oxygen therapy (to achieve a saturation of 88–92%) is the basis for treating respiratory insufficiency in COPD. However, if respiratory acidosis develops or progresses (pH < 7.35) during careful monitoring of this treatment, NIV is recommended [7, 23].

4.2.2 Examinations and procedures before the start of the NIV

Examinations before the start of NIV are recommended the same as in Section 3.2.2. A chest radiograph is necessary to determine whether the deterioration of the patient's condition is caused by pneumothorax or pulmonary edema.

4.2.3 Management of NIV in an obese patient with AECOPD

A patient with AECOPD with respiratory acidosis is at extreme risk of early death, and early intervention is necessary [59]. NIV is highly effective in this indication but does not replace the standard treatment of AECOPD, which must be given in each case. NIV should be started as soon as it is confirmed that regulated oxygen therapy is failing. In the case of AECOPD, as in the case of OHS, CPAP is not an appropriate treatment (as respiratory support). The method of choice is bilevel ventilation [7, 17, 23]. In treating obese patients with COPD, we can generally proceed from the procedures in OHS, with certain specifics for airway disorder.

4.2.3.1 Important notations on the management of NIV in obese patients with AECOPD

- **Interface**: Since mouth breathing predominates in AECOPD, we prefer the oronasal (full-face) mask. Prevention of skin lesions is necessary, and mask rotation is useful. In case of failure to use the mask, helmet ventilation may be a suitable alternative.

- **Humidification**: Humidified ventilatory circuits are necessary for patients with airway disease.

- **Ventilation mode**: Spontaneous-timed (ST), pressure-controlled (PC) mode, allowing you to set the backup frequency.

- **EPAP**: For COPD, it is standardly recommended to set EPAP to exceed intrinsic PEEP in the airways (usually 5–6 cm H_2O). Because obese patients with COPD have a high risk of OSA, it is necessary to proceed as in the diagnosis of OHS and increase EPAP to eliminate upper airway obstruction (which is a condition for successful NIV).

- **IPAP**: The inspiratory pressure settings are like those in an acute patient with OHS. The purpose is to ensure sufficient pressure support, unloading of respiratory muscles, and reduction of respiratory work. It is necessary to achieve the required tidal volume, chest excursions, decrease respiratory rate, and eliminate the diaphragmatic paradox. IPAP can start at 15 cm H_2O, titrates upwards gradually in the range of 20–30, which are commonly used to manage AECOPD (mostly in pH < 7.25) [17, 44, 60]. However, patient tolerance is fundamental, and pressure increases must be gradual and monitored.

- **Ensuring the target volume**: Using ventilation pressure-controlled modes with target tidal volume settings can be useful, well-tolerated, and effective in managing AECOPD in obese patients. In addition, from a practical point of view, in an acute state, automatic modes (e.g., AVAPS™, target volume) require less intervention by staff (in terms of parameter titration) than in simple bilevel modes. In COPD, tidal volume can be targeted at 6 (maximum 8) mL kg^{-1} ideal body weight [60]. The rate of pressure change (to adjust tidal volume) is suitable to choose medium to fast (in super-obese patients).

- **Backup rate**: Backup respiratory rate should be set at 15 breaths/min [23].

- **Inspiratory time**: For mandatory breaths, 0.8–1.2 s according to breathing frequency. I-E ratio can be set 1:2–1:3 [20, 23]. For ventilators with the possibility of setting the inspiratory ramp and rise time, it is advisable to set them so that the patient has enough time to inhale and, in the case of prolonged expiration, allow him/her to exhale effectively.

- **Oxygen**: Standardly added to the ventilation circuit to achieve a saturation of 88–92%.

- **Monitoring choices and contraindications to NIV** are the same as in OHS (Section 3.2.3).

4.2.3.2 Failure of acute NIV and indication of endotracheal intubation in AECOPD

Predictors of NIV failure have already been mentioned in Section 3.2.3. The documented percentage of NIV failure ranges widely from 5 to 40% (depending on the predictors of failure, patient selection, and staff experience with NIV). Analysis of several studies has shown that the most significant predictor of NIV failure is pH 1 h after the onset of NIV, followed by the severity of the underlying disease and patient compliance [61]. If the pH after 1–2 h of NIV is below 7.25, respiratory rate > 25/min, or new confusion or distress appears, consider intubation [17]. Nevertheless, if NIV adds to patient distress and intubation has been inappropriate, NIV should be discontinued, and palliative care measures adopted [17].

In case of NIV failure and planning for escalation of treatment to invasive mechanical ventilation (IMV), it is necessary to [23, 60]:

- monitor and document parameters and signs indicating intubation

- document and provide a decision in "do not intubate" patients

- discuss the management with the patient and family

- plan intubation before late failure of NIV

4.2.4 Further recommendations after successful acute ventilation in COPD

NIV may be an appropriate option in patients who have survived intubation and invasive mechanical ventilation and require continued treatment for chronic respiratory failure. However, in ventilator-dependent patients requiring ventilation for 12 h or more, tracheostomy may be considered and is highly recommended if the ventilation time exceeds 16 h per day. In this case, it is necessary to provide a ventilation device with an integrated battery [17, 40]. There are at least two reasons why we can assume that patients who have survived AECOPD with a need for NIV or IMV will be candidates for long-term home ventilation. The first is that obese patients with COPD have probable or known sleep-disordered breathing and will require some form of PAP treatment [53, 56]. Secondly, an episode of acute hypercapnic respiratory failure (AHRF) is a milestone in the course of the disease that predicts adverse development and prognosis [17]. In contrast to OHS (where weight reduction can reverse the course of the disease), this fact supports the planning of long-term ventilation treatment in obese patients with COPD. Therefore, clinicians should discuss the management of possible future episodes of AHRF with patients following an episode requiring ventilatory support because there is a high risk of recurrence [17]. Timing of indications for home mechanical ventilation (HMV) in COPD is a debated topic and ultimately depends on the decision of the patient and the physician. If the patient's condition after AHRF is stable, does not require continued ventilation, he/she may be discharged from the hospital with a scheduled early follow-up. It is recommended to reassess postacute NIV COPD patients 2–4 weeks after clinical recovery. NIV should be considered if the pCO_2 remains >7 kPa (53 mm Hg) [47] or if sleep-disordered breathing is detected in a sleep study.

4.3 Ventilation strategies in stable obese COPD patients

COPD is a disease associated with a high risk of developing chronic respiratory insufficiency [41]. Despite long-standing discussions about whether long-term NIV can affect the course and prognosis of the disease, the reality is that more than a third of patients treated are patients with lung and airways diseases [62]. Moreover, we now know that long-term NIV positively affects the quality of life and symptoms and improves survival [46, 47]. Thus, the question is not whether to ventilate COPD patients, but which COPD patients benefit from NIV and when it should be initiated.

4.3.1 Overlap syndrome COPD-OSA

Obese patients with COPD are very likely to have OSA simultaneously, commonly referred to as overlap syndrome [63]. The prevalence of these diseases in the general population is up to 10%, but in severely ill patients with COPD, the prevalence of OSA may be much higher, especially in the obese [53]. The coexistence of both diseases leads to a combination of continuous hypoxia (due to COPD) and chronic intermittent hypoxia (during sleep in apnea episodes due to OSA) in patients, which contributes to the development of the described clinical phenotype (Section 4.1) [57]. CPAP is the standard treatment for OSA and overlap syndrome [64]. However, CPAP treatment alone is more suitable for normocapnic patients with COPD, as it may not be effective in reversing hypoventilation and hypoxemia. Options should be carefully considered, and if nocturnal hypoxemia persists despite CPAP treatment, NIV may be an appropriate treatment instead of adding oxygen therapy to CPAP. In COPD patients diagnosed with OSA in the sleep laboratory, CPAP has been shown to fail in more than one-fifth. Although there are no clear limits to the efficacy of CPAP, treatment failure and NIV indication are more common in patients who are more obese, have worse lung function, hypercapnia, and more severe hypoxemia (with a longer desaturation time below 90% during nocturnal PSG) [65].

4.3.2 Indications for NIV in chronic hypercapnic respiratory failure in COPD

There is not only one criterion for indicating long-term NIV in COPD, which is confirmed by common practice that patients need to be approached individually [7, 9, 44, 66]. Long-term NIV may be indicated at a stable stage of COPD or after overcoming an acute exacerbation, meeting specific criteria, and considering the patient's needs. An important factor influencing the decision on the need for NIV is the presence of OSA. Contrary to the diagnosis of OHS with severe OSA, in the case of COPD-OSA overlap and hypercapnia, CPAP is not an appropriate option. CPAP may be effective in normocapnia in this case, but in hypercapnic COPD and the likelihood of progression of the underlying lung disease, NIV is the treatment of choice.

Long-term NIV may be indicated in well-established COPD (treated according to guidelines) in which there are persistent symptoms of chronic hypoventilation (hypercapnia), **and at least one of the following criteria is met:**

- chronic daytime $PaCO_2 > 50$ mm Hg
- nocturnal hypercapnia with $PaCO_2 > 55$ mm Hg
- daytime hypercapnia with $PaCO_2$ 45–50 mm Hg and nocturnal rise in transcutaneous CO_2 ($PTCCO_2$) ≥ 10 mm Hg
- stable daytime hypercapnia with $PaCO_2$ 45–50 mm Hg and at least two hospitalizations for hypercapnic respiratory failure within the past 12 months
- overlap syndrome COPD-OSA and daytime hypercapnia with $PaCO_2 > 45$ mm Hg
- after overcoming an acute exacerbation, if the need for respiratory support persists (based on clinical estimation)

4.3.3 Examinations before the start of long-term NIV

Blood gas collection and chest X-ray are recommended as standard. If possible, it is advisable to carry out a sleep study, preferably with the measurement of transcutaneous capnometry. Finally, the examination of lung functions is critical. Although this is not indicated directly in COPD exacerbation, in patients with a controversial diagnosis (especially in an obese patient), a misdiagnosis of COPD is common. Planning spirometry and possible body plethysmography with a distance from exacerbation before setting for long-term NIV will make it possible to clarify the diagnosis and set up treatment effectively.

4.3.4 Management of long-term NIV

Because patients with COPD form a wide range of different phenotypes, making precise recommendations on setting long-term NIV is not easy. In recent years, various approaches have been used, including the so-called low-intensity NIV (LI-NIV) and high-intensity NIV (HI-NIV) [44, 66]. The main difference is that HI-NIV uses higher values of IPAP and backup frequency to achieve normocapnia [48]. This approach has been shown in clinical trials to be effective in improving symptoms and quality of life and even in improving survival [45–47]. NIV was most effective in those COPD patients where IPAP over 18 cm H_2O was used, baseline $paCO_2$ was over 55 mm Hg, and NIV was used overnight for more than 5 h [44]. Another option is to use volume-targeted ventilation modes. In COPD, their use is equally effective compared to HI-NIV [67]. It can make sense to obese patients with COPD because they allow them to better adapt to current and later patient needs when set up correctly.

4.3.4.1 Important notes on the management of long-term NIV in obese patients with COPD

- **Interface**: The choice of mask for long-term NIV is at the patient's and the physician's discretion but must ensure adequate ventilation and low leakage (e.g., in mouth breathers).

- **Ventilation modes and pressure settings**: Spontaneous-timed (ST) is the best option for long-term NIV. Automatic modes can be used to titrate settings, especially EPAP. The pressure setting is similar to AECOPD; the aim is to ensure airway patency (eliminate obstructive apnea). IPAP titration in chronic respiratory insufficiency may be less steep than in acute conditions. We can start at IPAP 12 cm H_2O and gradually increase above 18 cm H_2O (often between 20 and 30). We titrate the backup frequency slightly higher than in OHS. However, the basis is to ensure patient tolerance and compliance. Target volume modes can be used in obese patients like in AECOPD.

- **Oxygen**: In hypercapnic COPD, inhalation of oxygen through a nasal cannula is risky due to the progression of hypoventilation. If the NIV alone is insufficient to maintain saturation above 90%, it is advisable to add oxygen to the ventilation circuit.

5. Conclusion

This chapter aimed to discuss different approaches to the treatment of respiratory failure depending on the situation and diagnosis in obese patients. Up-to-date information from evidence-based medicine and international guidelines was used in the preparation of the chapter. Although COPD and OHS are different diagnoses with different prognoses, in obese patients, they are associated with the presence of sleep-disordered breathing. It is obstructive sleep apnea that seems to be a key factor contributing to the clinical picture of the so-called obese patient with COPD, and early diagnosis and treatment can reverse the negative impact of the disease on patients' health.

Author details

Pavol Pobeha
Department of Respiratory Medicine and Tuberculosis, Faculty of Medicine, P.J. Safarik University and L. Pasteur University Hospital, Kosice, Slovakia

*Address all correspondence to: pavol.pobeha@upjs.sk

References

[1] Chooi YC, Ding C, Magkos F. The epidemiology of obesity. Metabolism. 2019;**92**:6-10. DOI: 10.1016/j.metabol.2018.09.005. Epub 2018 Sep 22

[2] Pépin JL, Timsit JF, Tamisier R, Borel JC, Lévy P, Jaber S. Prevention and care of respiratory failure in obese patients. The Lancet Respiratory Medicine. 2016;**4**(5):407-418. DOI: 10.1016/S2213-2600(16)00054-0

[3] Malli F, Papaioannou AI, Gourgoulianis KI, Daniil Z. The role of leptin in the respiratory system: An overview. Respiratory Research. 2010;**11**(1):152. DOI: 10.1186/1465-9921-11-152

[4] Rivas E, Arismendi E, Agustí A, Sanchez M, Delgado S, Gistau C, et al. Ventilation/perfusion distribution abnormalities in morbidly obese subjects before and after bariatric surgery. Chest. 2015;**147**(4):1127-1134. DOI: 10.1378/chest.14-1749

[5] Peppard PE, Young T, Barnet JH, Palta M, Hagen EW, Hla KM. Increased prevalence of sleep-disordered breathing in adults. American Journal of Epidemiology. 2013;**177**(9):1006-1014. DOI: 10.1093/aje/kws342. Epub 2013 Apr 14

[6] Elliot JG, Donovan GM, Wang KCW, Green FHY, James AL, Noble PB. Fatty airways: Implications for obstructive disease. The European Respiratory Journal. 2019;**54**(6):1900857. DOI: 10.1183/13993003.00857-2019

[7] Nava S, Fanfulla F, editors. Non-Invasive Artificial Ventilation—How, When and Why. Italia: Springer-Verlag; 2010. 190 p. DOI: 10.1007/978-88-470-5526-1

[8] McKim DA, Road. J, Avendano M, Abdool S, Cote F, Duguid N, Fraser J, Maltais F, Morrison DL, O'Connell C, Petrof BJ, Rimmer K, Skomro R. Canadian Thoracic Society Home Mechanical Ventilation Committee. Home mechanical ventilation: A Canadian Thoracic Society clinical practice guideline. Canadian Respiratory Journal. 2011;**18**(4):197-215. DOI: 10.1155/2011/139769

[9] Windisch W, Walterspacher S, Siemon K, Geiseler J, Sitter H. German Society for Pneumology. Guidelines for non-invasive and invasive mechanical ventilation for treatment of chronic respiratory failure. Published by the German Society for Pneumology (DGP). Pneumologie. 2010;**64**(10):640-652. DOI: 10.1055/s-0030-1255558. Epub 2010 Aug 26

[10] Mokhlesi B, Kryger MH, Grunstein RR. Assessment and management of patients with obesity hypoventilation syndrome. Proceedings of the American Thoracic Society. 2008;**5**:218-225. DOI: 10.1513/pats.200708-122MG

[11] Mokhlesi B. Obesity hypoventilation syndrome: A state-of-the-art review. Respiratory Care. 2010;**55**(10):1347-1362, discussion 1363-1365

[12] Marik PE, Chen C. The clinical characteristics and hospital and post-hospital survival of patients with the obesity hypoventilation syndrome: Analysis of a large cohort. Obesity Science and Practice. 2016;**2**(1):40-47. DOI: 10.1002/osp4.27. Epub 2016 Feb 9

[13] Scott S, Currie J, Albert P, Calverley P, Wilding JPH. Risk of misdiagnosis, health-related quality of life, and BMI in patients who are overweight with doctor-diagnosed asthma. Chest. 2012;**141**(3):616-624. DOI: 10.1378/chest.11-0948. Epub 2011 Aug 25

[14] Masa JF, Pépin JL, Borel JC, Mokhlesi B, Murphy PB,

Sánchez-Quiroga MÁ. Obesity hypoventilation syndrome. European Respiratory Review. 2019;**28**(151): 180097. DOI: 10.1183/16000617.0097-2018

[15] Hart N, Murphy P. Chronic NIV in OHS. In: Simonds A, editor. Handbook of Non-Invasive Ventilation, ERS Practical. Sheffield: European Respiratory Society; 2015. pp. 197-203. DOI: 10.1183/9781849840767.eph01

[16] Ramírez-Molina VR, Gómez-de-Terreros FJ, Barca-Durán J, Masa JF. Non-invasive positive airway pressure in obesity hypoventilation syndrome and chronic obstructive pulmonary disease: Present and future perspectives. COPD. 2017;**14**(4):418-428. DOI: 10.1080/15412555.2017.1317730 Epub 2017 May 9

[17] Davidson AC, Banham S, Elliott M, Kennedy D, Gelder C, Glossop A, et al. BTS/ICS guideline for the ventilatory management of acute hypercapnic respiratory failure in adults. Thorax. 2016;**71**(Suppl. 2):ii1-ii35. DOI: 10.1136/thoraxjnl-2015-208209. Erratum in: Thorax. 2017;**72**(6):588

[18] Patout M, Gagnadoux F, Rabec C, Trzepizur W, Georges M, Perrin C, et al. AVAPS-AE versus ST mode: A randomized controlled trial in patients with obesity hypoventilation syndrome. Respirology. 2020;**25**(10):1073-1081. DOI: 10.1111/resp.13784. Epub 2020 Feb 13

[19] Ambrogio C, Lowman X, Kuo M, Malo J, Prasad AR, Parthasarathy S. Sleep and non-invasive ventilation in patients with chronic respiratory insufficiency. Intensive Care Medicine. 2009;**35**(2):306-313. DOI: 10.1007/s00134-008-1276-4. Epub 2008 Sep 16

[20] Ghosh D, Elliott MW. Acute non-invasive ventilation—Getting it right on the acute medical take. Clinical Medicine (London, England). 2019;**19**(3):237-242. DOI: 10.7861/clinmedicine.19-3-237

[21] Hollier CA, Harmer AR, Maxwell LJ, Menadue C, Willson GN, Unger G, et al. Moderate concentrations of supplemental oxygen worsen hypercapnia in obesity hypoventilation syndrome: A randomized crossover study. Thorax. 2014;**69**(4):346-353. DOI: 10.1136/thoraxjnl-2013-204389. Epub 2013 Nov 19

[22] Schönhofer B, Kuhlen R, Neumann P, Westhoff M, Berndt C, Sitter H. Clinical practice guideline: Non-invasive mechanical ventilation as treatment of acute respiratory failure. Deutsches Ärzteblatt International. 2008;**105**(24):424-433. DOI: 10.3238/arztebl.2008.0424. Epub 2008 Jun 13

[23] Elliot M. The patients with an acute hypercapnic exacerbation of COPD. In: Simonds A, editor. Handbook of Non-Invasive Ventilation, ERS Practical. Sheffield: European Respiratory Society; 2015. pp. 41-46. DOI: 10.1183/9781849840767.eph01

[24] Nicolini A, Lemyze M, Esquinas A, Barlascini C, Cavalleri MA. Predictors of non-invasive ventilation failure in critically ill obese patients: A brief narrative review. Advances in Respiratory Medicine. 2017;**85**(5):264-270. DOI: 10.5603/ARM.a2017.0044. Epub 2017 Oct 30

[25] Lemyze M, Taufour P, Duhamel A, Temime J, Nigeon O, Vangrunderbeeck N, et al. Determinants of non-invasive ventilation success or failure in morbidly obese patients in acute respiratory failure. PLoS One. 2014;**9**(5):e97563. DOI: 10.1371/journal.pone.0097563

[26] Mokhlesi B, Masa JF, Brozek JL, Gurubhagavatula I, Murphy PB, Piper AJ, et al. Evaluation and management of obesity hypoventilation syndrome. An official american thoracic

society clinical practice guideline. American Journal of Respiratory and Critical Care Medicine. 2019;**200**(3):e6-e24. DOI: 10.1164/rccm.201905-1071ST. Erratum in: American Journal of Respiratory and Critical Care Medicine. 2019;**200**(10):1326

[27] Piper AJ, Wang D, Yee BJ, Barnes DJ, Grunstein RR. Randomized trial of CPAP vs bilevel support in the treatment of obesity hypoventilation syndrome without severe nocturnal desaturation. Thorax. 2008;**63**(5):395-401. DOI: 10.1136/thx.2007.081315. Epub 2008 Jan 18

[28] Howard ME, Piper AJ, Stevens B, Holland AE, Yee BJ, Dabscheck E, et al. A randomized controlled trial of CPAP versus non-invasive ventilation for initial treatment of obesity hypoventilation syndrome. Thorax. 2017;**72**(5):437-444. DOI: 10.1136/thoraxjnl-2016-208559. Epub 2016 Nov 15

[29] Masa JF, Corral J, Alonso ML, Ordax E, Troncoso MF, Gonzalez M, et al. Efficacy of different treatment alternatives for obesity hypoventilation syndrome. Pickwick study. American Journal of Respiratory and Critical Care Medicine. 2015;**192**(1):86-95. DOI: 10.1164/rccm.201410-1900OC

[30] Corral J, Mogollon MV, Sánchez-Quiroga MÁ, Gómez de Terreros J, Romero A, Caballero C, et al. Echocardiographic changes with non-invasive ventilation and CPAP in obesity hypoventilation syndrome. Thorax. 2018;**73**(4):361-368. DOI: 10.1136/thoraxjnl-2017-210642. Epub 2017 Nov 16

[31] Masa JF, Mokhlesi B, Benítez I, Gomez de Terreros FJ, Sánchez-Quiroga MÁ, Romero A, et al. Long-term clinical effectiveness of continuous positive airway pressure therapy versus non-invasive ventilation therapy in patients with obesity hypoventilation syndrome: A multicentre, open label, randomised controlled trial. Lancet. 2019;**393**(10182):1721-1732. DOI: 10.1016/S0140-6736(18)32978-7. Epub 2019 Mar 29

[32] Masa JF, Mokhlesi B, Benítez I, Mogollon MV, Gomez de Terreros FJ, Sánchez-Quiroga MÁ, et al. Echocardiographic changes with positive airway pressure therapy in obesity hypoventilation syndrome. Long-term pickwick randomized controlled clinical trial. American Journal of Respiratory and Critical Care Medicine. 2020;**201**(5):586-597. DOI: 10.1164/rccm.201906-1122OC

[33] Pobeha P, Paranicova I, Trojova I, Tkacova R, Joppa P. Acute hemodynamic effects of non-invasive ventilation in patients with obesity hypoventilation syndrome. Bratislavské Lekárske Listy. 2021;**122**(4):248-250. DOI: 10.4149/BLL_2021_040

[34] Masa JF, Mokhlesi B, Benítez I, Gómez de Terreros Caro FJ, Sánchez-Quiroga MÁ, Romero A, et al. Cost-effectiveness of positive airway pressure modalities in obesity hypoventilation syndrome with severe obstructive sleep apnoea. Thorax. 2020;**75**(6):459-467. DOI: 10.1136/thoraxjnl-2019-213622. Epub 2020b Mar 26

[35] Orfanos S, Jaffuel D, Perrin C, Molinari N, Chanez P, Palot A. Switch of non-invasive ventilation (NIV) to continuous positive airway pressure (CPAP) in patients with obesity hypoventilation syndrome: A pilot study. BMC Pulmonary Medicine. 2017;**17**(1):50. DOI: 10.1186/s12890-017-0391-9

[36] Lastra AC, Masa JF, Mokhlesi B. CPAP titration failure is not equivalent to long-term CPAP treatment failure in patients with obesity hypoventilation syndrome: A case series. Journal of Clinical Sleep Medicine.

2020;**16**(11):1975-1981. DOI: 10.5664/jcsm.8712

[37] Braganza MV, Hanly PJ, Fraser KL, Tsai WH, Pendharkar SR. Predicting CPAP failure in patients with suspected sleep hypoventilation identified on ambulatory testing. Journal of Clinical Sleep Medicine. 2020;**16**(9):1555-1565. DOI: 10.5664/jcsm.8616

[38] Salord N, Mayos M, Miralda RM, Farré A, Carreras M, Sust R, et al. Continuous positive airway pressure in clinically stable patients with mild-to-moderate obesity hypoventilation syndrome and obstructive sleep apnoea. Respirology. 2013;**18**(7):1135-1142. DOI: 10.1111/resp.12131

[39] Arellano-Maric MP, Hamm C, Duiverman ML, Schwarz S, Callegari J, Storre JH, et al. Obesity hypoventilation syndrome treated with non-invasive ventilation: Is a switch to CPAP therapy feasible? Respirology. 2020;**25**(4):435-442. DOI: 10.1111/resp.13704. Epub 2019 Oct 9

[40] Windisch W, Geiseler J, Simon K, Walterspacher S, Dreher M, On behalf of the Guideline Commission. German national guideline for treating chronic respiratory failure with invasive and non-invasive ventilation—Revised edition 2017: Part 2. Respiration. 2018;**96**(2):171-203. DOI: 10.1159/000488667. Epub 2018 Jun 26

[41] Halpin DMG, Criner GJ, Papi A, Singh D, Anzueto A, Martinez FJ, et al. Global initiative for the diagnosis, management, and prevention of chronic obstructive lung disease. The 2020 GOLD science committee report on COVID-19 and chronic obstructive pulmonary disease. American Journal of Respiratory and Critical Care Medicine. 2021;**203**(1):24-36. DOI: 10.1164/rccm.202009-3533SO

[42] Roussos C. The failing ventilatory pump. Lung. 1982;**160**(2):59-84. DOI: 10.1007/BF02719275

[43] Rochwerg B, Brochard L, Elliott MW, Hess D, Hill NS, Nava S, et al. Official ERS/ATS clinical practice guidelines: Non-invasive ventilation for acute respiratory failure. European Respiratory Journal. 2017;**50**(2):1602426. DOI: 10.1183/13993003.02426-2016

[44] Windish W, Storre J. The patients with an acute hypercapnic exacerbation of COPD. In: Simonds A, editor. Handbook of Non-Invasive Ventilation, ERS Practical. Sheffield: European Respiratory Society; 2015. pp. 190-196. DOI: 10.1183/9781849840767.eph01

[45] Budweiser S, Hitzl AP, Jörres RA, Heinemann F, Arzt M, Schroll S, et al. Impact of noninvasive home ventilation on long-term survival in chronic hypercapnic COPD: A prospective observational study. International Journal of Clinical Practice. 2007;**61**(9):1516-1522. DOI: 10.1111/j.1742-1241.2007.01427.x

[46] Köhnlein T, Windisch W, Köhler D, Drabik A, Geiseler J, Hartl S, et al. Non-invasive positive pressure ventilation for the treatment of severe stable chronic obstructive pulmonary disease: A prospective, multicentre, randomised, controlled clinical trial. The Lancet Respiratory Medicine. 2014;**2**(9):698-705. DOI: 10.1016/S2213-2600(14)70153-5. Epub 2014 Jul 24

[47] Murphy PB, Rehal S, Arbane G, Bourke S, Calverley PMA, Crook AM, et al. Effect of home noninvasive ventilation with oxygen therapy vs oxygen therapy alone on hospital readmission or death after an acute COPD exacerbation: A randomized clinical trial. Journal of the American Medical Association. 2017;**317**(21):2177-2186. DOI: 10.1001/jama.2017.4451

[48] van der Leest S, Duiverman ML. High-intensity non-invasive ventilation in stable hypercapnic COPD: Evidence

of efficacy and practical advice. Respirology. 2019;**24**(4):318-328. DOI: 10.1111/resp.13450. Epub 2018 Nov 30

[49] Miravitlles M, Soler-Cataluña JJ, Calle M, Molina J, Almagro P, Quintano JA, et al. Spanish guidelines for management of chronic obstructive pulmonary disease (GesEPOC) 2017. Pharmacological treatment of stable phase. Archivos de Bronconeumologia. 2017;**53**(6):324-335. English, Spanish. DOI: 10.1016/j.arbres.2017.03.018. Epub 2017 May 3

[50] Zatloukal J, Brat K, Neumannova K, Volakova E, Hejduk K, Kocova E, et al. Chronic obstructive pulmonary disease—Diagnosis and management of stable disease; a personalized approach to care, using the treatable traits concept based on clinical phenotypes. Position paper of the Czech Pneumological and Phthisiological Society. Biomedical Papers of the Medical Faculty of the University Palacky, Olomouc, Czech Republic. 2020;**164**(4):325-356. DOI: 10.5507/bp.2020.056

[51] Rutten EP, Calverley PM, Casaburi R, Agusti A, Bakke P, Celli B, et al. Changes in body composition in patients with chronic obstructive pulmonary disease: Do they influence patient-related outcomes? Annals of Nutrition & Metabolism. 2013;**63**(3):239-247. DOI: 10.1159/000353211. Epub 2013 Nov 7

[52] Zewari S, Vos P, van den Elshout F, Dekhuijzen R, Heijdra Y. Obesity in COPD: Revealed and unrevealed issues. COPD. 2017;**14**(6):663-673. DOI: 10.1080/15412555.2017.1383978

[53] Schreiber A, Cemmi F, Ambrosino N, Ceriana P, Lastoria C, Carlucci A. Prevalence and predictors of obstructive sleep apnea in patients with chronic obstructive pulmonary disease undergoing inpatient pulmonary rehabilitation. COPD. 2018;**15**(3):265-270. DOI: 10.1080/15412555.2018.1500533. Epub 2018 Sep 21

[54] Adler D, Dupuis-Lozeron E, Janssens JP, Soccal PM, Lador F, Brochard L, et al. Obstructive sleep apnea in patients surviving acute hypercapnic respiratory failure is best predicted by static hyperinflation. PLoS One. 2018;**13**(10):e0205669. DOI: 10.1371/journal.pone.0205669

[55] McNicholas WT. Chronic obstructive pulmonary disease and obstructive sleep apnea overlaps in pathophysiology, systemic inflammation, and cardiovascular disease. American Journal of Respiratory and Critical Care Medicine. 2009;**180**(8):692-700. DOI: 10.1164/rccm.200903-0347PP. Epub 2009 Jul 23

[56] Barnes PJ, Burney PG, Silverman EK, Celli BR, Vestbo J, Wedzicha JA, et al. Chronic obstructive pulmonary disease. Nature Reviews. Disease Primers. 2015;**1**:15076. DOI: 10.1038/nrdp.2015.76

[57] Pobeha P, Joppa P, Koblizek V. Obézny pacients CHOCHP—Nový či opomenutý fenotyp CHOCHP? [Obese patient with COPD—A new or overlooked phenotype of COPD?]. Studia Pneumologica et Phthiseologica. 2019;**79**(4):129-133. Available from: http://www.pneumologie.cz/cislo/1542/4-2019/?potvrzeni1=1&potvrzeni2=1&potvrdit=ANO%0D%0A%0D%0A++++Vstoupit# [Accessed: 16 May 2021

[58] Nava S, Navalesi P, Conti G. Time of non-invasive ventilation. Intensive Care Medicine. 2006;**32**(3):361-370. DOI: 10.1007/s00134-005-0050-0. Epub 2006 Feb 14

[59] Wilkinson TM, Donaldson GC, Hurst JR, Seemungal TA, Wedzicha JA. Early therapy improves outcomes of exacerbations of chronic obstructive pulmonary disease. American Journal of Respiratory and Critical Care Medicine. 2004;**169**(12):1298-1303. DOI: 10.1164/rccm.200310-1443OC

[60] Sanchez D, Smith G, Piper A, Rolls K, On behalf of the Guideline development network members. Non-Invasive Ventilation Guidelines for Adult Patients with Acute Respiratory Failure: A Clinical Practice Guideline. Chatswood NSW: Agency for Clinical Innovation NSW Government Version 1; 2014. ISBN 978-1-74187-954-4. Available from: https://aci.health.nsw.gov.au/__data/assets/pdf_file/0007/239740/ACI14_Man_NIV_1-2.pdf [Accessed: 21 May 2021]

[61] Nava S, Ceriana P. Causes of failure of non-invasive mechanical ventilation. Respiratory Care. 2004;**49**(3):295-303

[62] Lloyd-Owen SJ, Donaldson GC, Ambrosino N, Escarabill J, Farre R, Fauroux B, et al. Patterns of home mechanical ventilation use in Europe: Results from the Eurovent survey. The European Respiratory Journal. 2005;**25**(6):1025-1031. DOI: 10.1183/09031936.05.00066704

[63] McNicholas WT. Chronic obstructive pulmonary disease and obstructive sleep apnoea-the overlap syndrome. Journal of Thoracic Disease. 2016;**8**(2):236-242. DOI: 10.3978/j.issn.2072-1439.2016.01.52

[64] Owens RL, Malhotra A. Sleep-disordered breathing and COPD: The overlap syndrome. Respiratory Care. 2010;**55**(10):1333-1344, discussion 1344-1346

[65] Kuklisova Z, Tkacova R, Joppa P, Wouters E, Sastry M. Severity of nocturnal hypoxia and daytime hypercapnia predicts CPAP failure in patients with COPD and obstructive sleep apnea overlap syndrome. Sleep Medicine. 2017;**30**:139-145. DOI: 10.1016/j.sleep.2016.02.012. Epub 2016 May 6

[66] Orr JE, Azofra AS, Tobias LA. Management of chronic respiratory failure in chronic obstructive pulmonary disease: High-intensity and low-intensity ventilation. Sleep Medicine Clinics. 2020;**15**(4):497-509. DOI: 10.1016/j.jsmc.2020.08.007

[67] Storre JH, Matrosovich E, Ekkernkamp E, Walker DJ, Schmoor C, Dreher M, et al. Home mechanical ventilation for COPD: High intensity versus target volume non-invasive ventilation. Respiratory Care. 2014;**59**(9):1389-1397. DOI: 10.4187/respcare.02941. Epub 2014 Jul 29

Chapter 5

Mechanical Ventilation in Neurocritical Patients

Thierry Hernández-Gilsoul, Jose de Jesús Vidal-Mayo and Alan Alexis Chacon-Corral

Abstract

Patients under neurocritical care may require mechanical ventilation for airway protection; respiratory failure can occur simultaneously or be acquired during the ICU stay. In this chapter, we will address the ventilatory strategies, in particular the role of protective lung ventilation, and the potential increase in intracranial pressure as a result of permissive hypercapnia, high airway pressures during recruitment maneuvers, and/or prone position. We will also describe some strategies to achieve mechanical ventilation liberation, including evaluation for tracheostomy, timing of tracheostomy, mechanical ventilation modalities for weaning and extubation, or tracheostomy weaning for mechanical ventilation.

Keywords: mechanical ventilation, neurocritical

1. Introduction

Neurological critically ill patients represent an important group in the intensive care unit (ICU) worldwide. About 20% of these patients require mechanical ventilation (MV) of which 20–25% will develop acute respiratory distress syndrome (ARDS) [1, 2]. Ventilatory management is controversial in this kind of population due to the complexity of the event and singularity of each case with acute brain injury (ABI). This includes traumatic brain injury (TBI), intracerebral hemorrhage (ICH), aneurysmatic subarachnoid hemorrhage (aSH), acute ischemic stroke (AIS), and other entities associated with high intracranial pressure (ICP). Additionally, brain damage may be prevented by avoiding pulmonary and systemic injury associated with mechanical ventilation. Thus, this topic is particularly important, since respiratory failure is the most frequent extracerebral organic failure in patients with ABI [3].

Recently, the VENTILA group reported some interesting characteristics, in the evolution of the ventilatory management in neurological critically ill patients, in three cohorts of patients with mechanical ventilation (2004, 2010, and 2016) [4]. In this multicentric international report of 4152 patients, the main pathologies were intracerebral hemorrhage and traumatic brain injury. One of the main results was an increment in the use of lung protective ventilation through time (47% in 2004, 63% in 2010 vs 65% in 2016; $p<0.001$). However, there were no differences in other outcomes such as length of stay in ICU, length of stay in hospital, mortality in the ICU, and mortality in the hospital. Some variables were associated with mortality in multivariate analyses such as age > 75 years old (OR 1.80, CI 95% 1.40–2.30),

SAPS II (Simplified Acute Physiology Score II) > 50 points (OR 2.31, CI 95% 1.87–2.86), occurrence of organic failure within the first 48 h after ABI (OR 1.79, IC 95% 1.59–2.0), and etiology of ABI, specifically TBI (OR 1.8, CI 95% 1.4–2.3), ischemic stroke (OR 3.94, CI 95% 2.47–6.31), and cerebral hemorrhage (OR 3.96, CI 95% 2.59–6.06).

2. Brain-lung cross talking

Acute brain injury can create issues in lung function and vice versa. This bidirectional brain-lung interaction is supported in experimental models and basic studies in humans, which have shown several neuroinflammatory, autonomic, immunologic, and endocrine pathways [5]. According to the so-called two-stroke model, when ACL occurs, a lung injury associated with systemic inflammation due to a "catecholamine storm" appears, first hit; subsequently these events can trigger an increase in permeability into the pulomnary capillaries, vasoconstriction in the pulmonary arterioles and recruitment of inflammatory cells in the alveoli, second hit [6].

Hypoxemia and hypercapnia are associated with lung injury and amplify acute brain injury. Both situations reduce cerebral vascular resistance, which consequently raises cerebral blood flow and increases ICP. Also, they can increase the systemic inflammatory response and produce extracerebral organic failures. In the literature, this chain of events had been denominated *dangerous cross talk* [7, 8]. Thus, ventilatory management has been considered a strategy to avoid ventilator-induced lung injury (VILI) through the use of lung-protective ventilation.

3. Ventilatory management

The most recent guidelines related to this topic are provided by the European Society of Intensive Care Medicine [9]. Evidence about most of these recommendations remains at a low level; for this reason, we present the most general suggestions in order to give a safety and efficient ventilatory management to these patients.

3.1 Oxygenation and carbon dioxide (CO_2) targets

In patients with ABI, it is fundamental to guarantee an optimal oxygenation to avoid secondary brain injury [10]. It is recommended to target "normoxia" with a partial arterial pressure of oxygen (PaO_2) between 80-120 mmHg and or a peripheral oxygen saturation (SpO_2) of ≥95% in patients with or without intracranial hypertension [9, 11].

In addition, some evidence suggests that hyperoxia is an independent factor associated to greater mortality and outcomes driven by several mechanisms: vasoconstriction of brain arteries, synthesis of reactive oxygen species (ROS) and damage associated molecular patterns (DAMPs) [10]. In a clinical trial of patients with traumatic brain injury (TBI), which evaluated two oxygenation strategies (normobaric hyperoxia and normoxia), there were no differences in the hospital length of stay, but the modified Rankin scale at discharge and at 6 month follow-up was better in the normoxia group [12].

In relation to the minute ventilation settings (respiratory rate times tidal volume) to modify the CO_2 content of the blood, it is recommended to adjust the ventilation to maintain normal levels of arterial pressure of carbon dioxide ($PaCO_2$) between 35 and 45 mmHg. Traditionally, it was considered that patients with ABI (specially population with TBI) should be maintained with hyperventilation;

however, this situation can lead to cerebral vasoconstriction that can worsen cerebral tissue hypoxia and ischemia [13]. In a randomized clinical trial conducted by Muizelaar et al., it found that patients with TBI undergoing systematic hyperventilation ($PaCO_2$ 25 ± 2 mmHg) had poorer outcomes at 3 and 6 months' follow-up compared with the normocapnia group ($PaCO_2$ 35 ± 2 mmHg). Deleterious findings were also documented in head injury patients who were managed with hyperventilation plus tromethamine addition as buffer [14]. Transient hyperventilation ($PaCO_2$ 30–35 mmHg) is only recommended as a rescue maneuver in cases of brain herniation [9].

3.2 Tidal volume (Vt)

Ventilation with Vt between 6 and 8 ml/kg of predicted body weight is considered a standard of ventilatory treatment in patients with ARDS and its application in general in patients under invasive ventilatory support. However, historically, neurocritical patients have been excluded from clinical trials that have evaluated this ventilatory therapeutic strategy due to the potential increase in intracranial pressure caused by hypercapnia and increased intrathoracic pressures [15].

In a multicenter cohort study, it was found that an average Vt of 9 ml/kg of predicted weight was used in this group of patients [15]. Additionally, it has been described that the use of high Vt has been associated with the development of ARDS in these patients [16] while other observational studies have found no evidence of this association; instead, driving pressure was the only ventilatory variable associated with the development of ARDS [17]. Likewise, there is no consistent evidence that the use of a Vt by itself increases intracranial pressure [15, 18].

A recent multicenter prospective study that used a strategy of low Vt (less than 7 ml/kg), moderate PEEP (6–8 cmH_2O), and a protocol for early extubation was associated with more days free of mechanical ventilation and lower mortality at 90 days, with no serious adverse events associated with this intervention [19]. Condensing this information, the administration of Vt of 6–8 ml/kg is suggested to maintain a plateau pressure of less than 25 cmH_2O and a driving pressure of less than 15 cmH_2O [8, 11, 13].

3.3 Positive end expiratory pressure (PEEP)

Implementation of PEEP associated with low Vt in the pulmonary protective ventilation strategy has been associated with better clinical outcomes, even in patients without ARDS [20]. Its use has been a useful strategy in neurocritical patients where oxygenation and ventilation are essential. The PEEP level has been considered a potential indirect maneuver that increases ICP in a directly proportional way. This led Asehnoune et al. to study the use of PEEP and its effect on intracranial pressure, comparing PEEP levels less than or greater than 5 cmH_2O; no clinically significant differences of episodes of intracranial hypertension were seen [19]. Boone et al. analyzed 341 patients with ABI, in which nonsignificant effects of PEEP on ICP or cerebral perfusion pressure (CPP) were documented [21]. Furthermore, in a study of patients with aSH divided into groups according to respiratory compliance, those with decreased respiratory compliance (<45 ml/cmH_2O) did not show changes in the hemodynamic variables, including CPP at diverse levels of PEEP [22].

In another prospective study of 20 patients with TBI with brain-tissue oxygenation ($P_{bt}O_2$) monitorization, an increase in the level of PEEP from 5 to 10 cmH_2O (24.60 ± 6.84 to 26.55 ± 7.09; p = 0.0001) and from 10 to 15 cmH_2O (26.55 ± 7.09 to 29.05 ± 7.07; p = 0.0001) significantly increased $P_{bt}O_2$ in these patients, without significant changes in ICP or CPP [23].

Therefore, it is recommended to administer a sufficient PEEP (5–8 cmH_2O) to maintain adequate oxygenation. In cases where PEEP is greater than 10–15 cmH_2O, it is suggested that advanced neuromonitoring be used to adjust this variable optimally [11, 13, 24].

3.4 Prone positioning

Mechanical ventilation in the prone position is also a standard of treatment for patients with moderate-severe ARDS, since it reduces mortality in addition to improving oxygenation, respiratory mechanics, and ventilation-perfusion imbalance. However, due to the potential increase in ICP and reduction in CCP, these patients have also been excluded from clinical studies to evaluate this intervention [13].

In an observational study of patients with aSH, who fulfilled criteria for ARDS within the first 2 weeks, a significant increase in oxygenation was found (97.3 ± 20.7 mmHg in the supine position to 126.6 ± 31.7 mmHg in the prone position) as well as an increase in $P_{bt}O_2$ (26.8 ± 10.9 mmHg to 31.6 ± 12.2 mmHg; $p < 0.0001$) with a good tolerance of the intervention (prone position for 14 hours). In contrast to a concomitant increase in ICP and a decrease in CPP, however, overall, the benefit in systemic oxygenation was greater than the effects on cerebral perfusion and intracranial pressure [25].

In the same way, other observational studies have reported that this maneuver improves patient oxygenation and $P_{bt}O_2$ with a tendency to increase ICP but without reducing CPP. One report with 8 patients showed a significant increase in oxygenation with an increase in ICP and CPP as well as an improvement in $P_{bt}O_2$ [26]. Roth et al. found in a retrospective study that patients had a significant increase in oxygenation with an increase in ICP without significant changes in CPP [27].

Recommendations in this group of patients suggest ventilation in the prone position. In patients with moderate-severe ARDS without evidence of intracranial hypertension, it is a safe and effective strategy. However, the risks and benefits of the intervention should be considered, and the patient must have multimodal monitoring to determine the effects on both systemic and cerebral hemodynamics and oxygenation [9, 11].

3.5 Alveolar recruitment maneuvers

Another controversial aspect is the use of alveolar recruitment maneuvers, due to the potential risk of increasing intracranial pressure with reduction of CPP [13]. In systematic reviews and meta-analysis of ARDS studies, it was found that this intervention is associated with an improvement in the oxygenation of patients but without effects in other outcomes such as mortality or duration of mechanical ventilation [28, 29].

In studies carried out in this population, conflicting results have been found regarding the efficacy of this intervention to improve oxygenation; however, regarding neurological variables, some studies described an increase in ICP associated with a decrease in CPP without improvement in oxygenation [30, 31]; another study found that recruitment maneuvers significantly affected cerebral hemodynamics [32].

Although the most recent guidelines for ventilatory management of these patients do not issue any recommendation due to limited evidence [9], expert recommendations suggest that this intervention can be considered individually in patients with acute brain injury and concomitant ARDS with an invasive neuro-monitoring for the potential risks and benefits of these maneuvers [8, 13].

4. Extracorporeal life support (ECLS)

Extracorporeal membrane oxygenation ventilation (ECMO) and extracorporeal CO_2 removal ($ECCO_2R$) have gained popularity for patients with hypoxemic respiratory failure refractory to conventional ventilation strategies; however, because the evidence for this intervention is anecdotal in this patient population [33, 34] and there is a risk of catastrophic complications in patients with ABI (especially intracranial hemorrhage due to the need for routine anticoagulation), there is no consensus to carry out this intervention in neurocritical patients [9, 11, 13]. Heparin-free regional citrate anticoagulation, like in renal replacement circuits, may offer an alternative to this problem [35]. The use of regional citrate anticoagulation continuous veno-venous hemofiltration (RCA-CVVH) connected to an ECMO circuit, with low heparin or heparin-free ECMO, has been reported [36].

In an experimental model of severe hypercapnic acidosis, regional anticoagulation with citrate solution achieved the anticoagulation goal as well as standard heparin anticoagulation but did not improve CO_2 removal and led to more hypocalcemia and hypotension [37].

5. Weaning from mechanical ventilation

Historically, the population of neurocritical patients has been considered at high risk of failure to extubation (from 10 to 38% failure), and hence there is delayed withdrawal of mechanical ventilation which is associated with higher rates of ventilator associated pneumonia (VAP) and airway injury; longer mechanical ventilation and ICU length stay, and higher mortality [15, 38, 39].

The recommendations of the international guidelines for the withdrawal of mechanical ventilation do not contemplate specific aspects for this population [40, 41], in addition to the fact that certain general aspects of these consensuses are not applicable for neurocritical patients:

- The process by which the patient is on mechanical ventilation is not resolved in most cases of patients with ABI [3, 39, 42].

- Evaluation of the state of consciousness (and, therefore, the ability to follow commands) is altered in a significant proportion of patients. In addition, scales used for the neurological evaluation in neurocritical patients on mechanical ventilation do not precisely discriminate success versus failure after extubation [40, 41]. Some studies have found that a score greater than 8 or greater than 10 in Glasgow Coma Scale (GCS) is associated with a successful withdrawal from mechanical ventilation [43, 44], while other series found that neither the GCS [42] nor the FOUR scale [45] was associated with successful extubation.

There is evidence that multidisciplinary and standardized protocols in these patients are associated with better outcomes and a higher rate of successful withdrawal from mechanical ventilation [46, 47]. One tool designed for this population is the VISAGE score by Asehnoune et al [44]. This score was derived from a multicenter prospective cohort that included a heterogeneous population of patients with ABI (n = 437), of which 77.3% had a successful extubation. From the multivariate analysis of the factors associated with successful extubation, 4 variables with significant association were found that made up the VISAGE score: visual pursuit, swallowing attempts, age under 40 years, and GCS greater than 10 points (**Table 1**). According to the original validation study, a score on this scale greater than or equal to 3 points

A score ≥ 3 is associated with 90% extubation success; each variable has a value of 1 point • Age < 40 years • Visual pursuit • Swallowing attempts • Glasgow coma score > 10 points
[44].

Table 1.
VISAGE score.

has a sensitivity of 62%, specificity of 79%, positive predictive value of 90%, negative predictive value of 39%, positive likelihood ratio of 2.9, and negative likelihood ratio of 0.5 to predict extubation success. This scale represents a practical tool for use in the patient's bed, for which several experts have recommended its clinical use; however, external validation in other patient cohorts is still pending [48, 49].

In a systematic review with meta-analysis, Wang et al. found that other variables associated with extubation failure in neurocritical patients are the presence of pneumonia, atelectasis, mechanical ventilation for more than 24 h, a score of GCS lower than 8 (OR = 4.96.95% CI = 1.61–15.26, p = 0.005), the inability to follow orders (OR = 2.07.95% CI = 1.15–3.71, p = 0.02), thick secretions, and alteration in cough reflex [50]. Another score that evaluates the ability to protect the airway has been proposed (the Airway score), which takes into consideration variables such as the amount and quality of respiratory secretions, gag and cough reflex, and patients with a score of less than 6 who are candidates for IMV withdrawal. Nevertheless, it should be considered that there is a wide variability in the qualitative assessment of respiratory secretions and that there is no extensive external validation of this tool [51].

Regarding the actual evidence of tracheostomy performance, it has been observed that intensivist achieves more frequently tracheostomies in neurocritical patients (up to 45%) compared to general patients in the ICU [52]. The theorical benefits of tracheostomy are that it decreases the work of breathing and improves patient comfort when compared to an endotracheal tube. Tracheal stoma that does not generate pain after 48–72 h of tracheostomy placement. Reduction or suspension of sedation and opioid analgesia, as well as less work of breathing are the theorical benefits that generate greater patient comfort. Contrary to general belief, there is no evidence that it decreases the frequency of tracheal stenosis associated with prolonged ventilation. Even more, an endotracheal cannula also requires the inflation of a balloon to isolate and protect the airway from bronchoaspiration; thus, tracheal stenosis is also a complication, which according to a case study is more complicated (infraglottic stenosis) and may not resolve more frequently compared to tracheal stenosis acquired with an orotracheal tube [53].

According to this information and consensus, it is recommended to consider to facilitate the withdrawal of mechanical ventilation in the following cases: infratentorial lesions, inability to protect the airway (inadequate management of respiratory secretions), altered central respiratory drive, slow or unfavorable neurological recovery, and patients with recurrent extubation failure.

However, the precise indications for its performance and the timing of the intervention remain poorly defined in the literature [38, 48, 54].

A highly controversial aspect is the performance of "early tracheostomy," which has been defined as placing it within the first 7 days [55] (there are reports that define it from day 5 to day 10) of mechanical ventilation [56, 57].

Large series of patients that have compared early versus late tracheostomy have not found a benefit in terms of mortality, although there is a trend of better outcomes in the early tracheostomy group, such as reduction in the frequency of ventilator-associated pneumonia, fewer days of mechanical ventilation, and a shorter length of stay in intensive care [58, 59]. In the SETPOINT study (Stroke-related Early Tracheostomy vs. Prolonged Orotracheal Intubation in Neurocritical care Trial) that randomized 60 patients with stroke or cerebral hemorrhage to early tracheostomy (day 1–3 of mechanical ventilation) versus standard tracheostomy (between 7 and 14 days), no difference was found in the primary endpoint, which was the length of stay in the ICU (median, interquartile range [IQR] 8, 16–28 days versus 17 [13–22] days, median difference: 1 [−2 to 6]; $p = 0.38$) although in the intervention group, mortality in the ICU and at 6 months was significantly lower (10 versus 14%; $p < 0.01$ and 27% versus 60% $p = 0.02$), without finding other differences in other secondary outcomes [60].

The CENTER-TBI study that was a prospective European multicenter cohort of adult patients with head trauma found that the factors associated with the decision to perform a tracheostomy were older age (HR = 1.04, 95% CI 1.01–1.07; $p = 0.003$), GCS less than or equal to 8 (HR = 1.70, 95% CI = 1.22–2.36 at 7; $p < 0.001$), thoracic trauma (HR = 1.24, 95% CI = 1.01–1.52, $p = 0.020$), hypoxemia (HR = 1.37, 95% CI = 1.05–1.79, $p = 0.048$), and absence of pupillary reactivity (HR = 1.76, 95% CI = 1.27–2.45 at 7; $p < 0.001$). Additionally, a wide heterogeneity was identified in the frequency (7.9–50.2%) and timing of early tracheostomy practice (0–17.6%) in

	Points
Neurological function	
Dysphagia (4 points)	4
Observed aspiration (3 points)	3
GCS on admission < 10 (3 points)	3
Neurological lesion	
Brain stem (4 points)	4
Ischemic stroke > 2/3 middle cerebral artery territory (4 points)	4
ICH volume > 25 ml (4 points)	4
Hydrocephalus (4 points)	4
Space-occupying cerebellar (3 points)	3
Diffuse lesion (3 points)	3
Extracerebral organ function-procedure	
APACHE II score > 20 (4 points)	4
Sepsis (3 points)	3
Additional respiratory disease (3 points)	3
$PaO_2/FiO_2 < 150$ (2 points)	2
LIS score > 1 (2 points)	2
Neurosurgical intervention (2 points)	2

A score > 8 in combination with an estimate of an experienced neurointensivist suggests prolonged ventilation and need of tracheostomy.
GCS = glasgow coma scale. ICH = intracerebral hemorrhage. PaO_2 = partial arterial pressure of oxygen. APACHE II = acute physiology and chronic health evaluation II. LIS = lung injury score.
[62, 63].

Table 2.
SET score to estimate tracheostomy need after severe stroke.

this cohort. Late tracheostomy (after 7 days) was associated with worse neurological outcomes and a longer stay in the intensive care unit [61].

In acute cerebrovascular events (ischemic stroke, cerebral hemorrhage, and aSH), a specific score for predicting tracheostomy has been designed and tested in these patients. The SET score (**Table 2**) that combines various variables from 3 items (neurological evaluation, characteristics of the injury, and extracerebral organic procedure/function) is the one with the greatest external validation for use in this population. A SET score of >10 points has a sensitivity of 64–81%, a specificity of 57–86%, and an area under the curve of 0.74 (95% CI 0.68–0.81) [62, 63].

In terms of an invasive procedure without complications, percutaneous tracheostomy is practically equivalent to surgical tracheostomy. Some systematic reviews with meta-analyses have found that the former has fewer stoma infections, with similar rates of bleeding and other procedural complications [64–66].

6. Conclusion

Neurocritical patients represent a particularly challenging subgroup for ventilatory management due to coexistence of acute brain injury associated with other organ failure, the most frequent being respiratory failure. Management of mechanical ventilation should prevent secondary brain injury by ensuring optimal ventilation and oxygenation. The use of additional strategies to standard management of pulmonary protective ventilation (high PEEP, recruitment maneuvers, and extracorporeal circulatory support) in patients with refractory respiratory failure should be individualized and be accompanied by advanced neuromonitoring (invasive measurement of intracranial pressure and cerebral tissue pressure oxygen). It is important to avoid a late withdrawal of mechanical ventilation using adjuvant scales such as the VISAGE score; theorical benefits from tracheostomy include reduction and suspension of sedation and opioid analgesia as well as patient comfort due to lower work of breathing and may be considered in patients with slow neurological recovery, failure to extubation, and those patients with dysphagia or altered state of consciousness resulting from a primary injury to the central nervous system.

Author details

Thierry Hernández-Gilsoul*, Jose de Jesús Vidal-Mayo
and Alan Alexis Chacon-Corral
Emergency Department, Instituto Nacional de Ciencias Médicas y Nutrición
Salvador Zubrian (INCMNSZ), Mexico City, Mexico

*Address all correspondence to: thierry.hernandezg@incmnsz.mx

References

[1] Esteban A, Anzueto A, Alia I, et al. How is mechanical ventilation employed in the intensive care unit? An international utilization review. American Journal of Respiratory and Critical Care Medicine. 2000; **161**:1450-1458

[2] Hoesch RE, Lin E, Young M, et al. Acute lung injury in critical neurological illness. Critical Care Medicine. 2012; **40**:587-593

[3] Zygun DA, Kortbeek JB, Fick GH, et al. Non-neurologic organ dysfunction in severe traumatic brain injury. Critical Care Medicine. 2005;**33**:654-660

[4] Tejerina EE, Pelosi P, Robba C, et al. Evolution over time of ventilatory management and outcome of patients with neurologic disease. Critical Care Medicine. 2021;**49**(7):1095-1106

[5] Stevens RD, Puybasset L. The brain-lung axis. Intensive Care Medicine. 2011;**37**:1054-1056

[6] Mascia L. Acute lung injury in patients with server brain injury: A double hit model. Neurocritical Care. 2011;**37**:1182-1191

[7] Pelosi P, Rocco PRM. The lung and the brain: A dangerous cross-talk. Critical Care. 2011;**15**:168

[8] Stevens RD, Piran P. Lung-protective ventilation and adjunctive strategies to manage respiratory failure: Are they safe in the neurological patient? Current Opinion in Critical Care. 2021; **27**:115-119

[9] Robba C, Poole D, McNett M, et al. Mechanical ventilation in patients with acute brain injury: Recommendations of the European Society of Intensive Care Medicine consensus. Intensive Care Medicine. 2020;**46**(12):2397-2410

[10] Vincent JL, Taccone FS, He X. Harmful effects of hyperoxia in postcardiac arrest, sepsis, traumatic brain injury, or stroke: The importance of individualized oxygen therapy in critically ill patients. Canadian Respiratory Journal. 2017;**2017**:2834956

[11] Frisvold SH, Robba C, Guérin C. What respiratory targets should be recommended in patients with brain injury and respiratory failure? Intensive Care Medicine. 2019;**45**:683-686

[12] Taber A, Pilehvari Z, Poorolajal J, Aghajanloo M. Effects of normobaric hyperoxia in traumatic brain injury: A randomized crontrolled clinical trial. Journal of Neurosurgery. 1991; **75**:731-739

[13] Battaglini D, Pelosi P, Robba C. Ten falses beliefs about mechanical ventilation in patients with brain injury. In: Vincent JL. (eds) Annual update in Intensive Care and Emergency Medicine 2020. Cham: Springer; 2020. p. 441-455. DOI: 10.1007/978-3-030-37323-8_34

[14] Muizelaar JP, Marmarou A, Ward JD, et al. Adverse effects of prolonged hyperventilation in patients with severe head injury: A randomized clinical trial. Journal of Neurosurgery. 1991;**75**(5):731-739

[15] Pelosi P, Ferguson ND, Frutos-Vivar F, et al. Management and outcome of mechanically ventilated neurologic patients. Critical Care Medicine. 2011;**39**:1482-1492

[16] Mascia L, Zavala E, Bosma K, et al. High tidal volume is associated with the development of acute lung injury after severe brain injury: An international observational study. Critical Care Medicine. 2007;**35**:1815 1820

[17] Tejerina E, Pelosi P, Muriel A, et al. Association between ventilatory settings and development of acute respiratory

distress syndrome in mechanically ventilated patients due to brain injury. Journal of Critical Care. 2017;**38**:341-345

[18] Ruggieri F, Beretta L, Corno L, et al. Feasibility of protective ventilation during elective supratentorial neurosurgery: A randomized, crossover, clinical trial. Journal of Neurosurgical Anesthesiology. 2018;**30**:246-250

[19] Asehnoune K, Mrozek S, Perrigault PF, et al. Amultifaceted strategy to reduce ventilation-associated mortality in brain-injured patients. The BI-VILI project: A nationwide quality improvement project. Intensive Care Medicine. 2017;**43**:957-970

[20] Serpa Neto A, Cardoso SO, Manetta JA, et al. Association between use of lung-protective ventilation with lower tidal volumes and clinical outcomes among patients without acute respiratory distress syndrome: A meta-analysis. Journal of the American Medical Association. 2012;**308**:1651-1659

[21] Boone MD, Jinadasa SP, Mueller A, et al. The effect of positive end-expiratory pressure on intracranial pressure and cerebral hemodynamics. Neurocritical Care. 2017;**26**:174-181

[22] Caricato A, Conti G, Della Corte F, et al. Effects of PEEP on the intracranial system of patients with head injury and subarachnoid hemorrhage: The role of respiratory system compliance. The Journal of Trauma. 2005;**58**:571-576

[23] Nemer SN, Caldeira JB, Santos RG, et al. Effects of positive end-expiratory pressure on brain tissue oxygen pressure of severe traumatic brain injury patients with acute respiratory distress syndrome: A pilot study. Journal of Critical Care. 2015;**30**:1263-1266

[24] Pérez NOR, Zamarrón LEI, Guerrero GMA, Deloya TE, Soriano OR, Sán-chez DJS, et al. PEEP: Dos lados de la misma moneda. Med Crit. 2021; **35**(1):34-46

[25] Reinprecht A, Greher M, Wolfsberger S, Dietrich W, Illievich UM, Gruber A. Prone position in subarachnoid hemorrhage patients with acute respiratory distress syndrome: Effects on cerebral tissue oxygenation and intracranial pressure. Critical Care Medicine. 2003;**31**:1831-1838

[26] Nekludov M, Bellander BM, Mure M. Oxygenation and cerebral perfusion pressure improved in the prone position. Acta Anaesthesiologica Scandinavica. 2006;**50**:932-936

[27] Roth C, Ferbert A, Deinsberger W, et al. Does prone positioning increase intracranial pressure? A retrospective analysis of patients with acute brain injury and acute respiratory failure. Neurocritical Care. 2014;**21**:186-191

[28] Hodgson C, Goligher E, Young M, et al. Recruitment manoeuvres for adults with acute respiratory distress syndrome. Cochrane Database of Systematic Reviews. 2016;**17**:CD006667

[29] Kang H, Yang H, Tong Z. Recruitment manoeuvres for adults with acute respiratory distress syndrome receiving mechanical ventilation: A systematic review and meta-analysis. Journal of Critical Care. 2019;**50**:1-10

[30] Bein T, Kuhr L-P, Bele S, Ploner F, Keyl C, Taeger K. Lung recruitment maneuver in patients with cerebral injury: Effects on intracranial pressure and cerebral metabolism. Intensive Care Medicine. 2002;**28**:554-558

[31] Flexman AM, Gooderham PA, Griesdale DE, Argue R, Toyota B. Effects of an alveolar recruitment maneuver on subdural pressure, brain swelling, and mean arterial pressure in patients undergoing supratentorial tumour resection: A randomized

crossover study. Canadian Journal of Anesthesia. 2017;**64**:626-633

[32] Zhang X, Yang Z, Wang Q, Fan H. Impact of positive end-expiratory pressure on cerebral injury patients with hypoxemia. The American Journal of Emergency Medicine. 2011;**29**:699-703

[33] Robba C, Ortu A, Bilotta F, et al. Extracorporeal membrane oxygenation for adult respiratory distress syndrome in trauma patients: A case series and systematic literature review. Journal of Trauma and Acute Care Surgery. 2017;**82**:165-173

[34] Unterberg M, Nowak H, Gottschalk A. Hypercapnic raised intracerebral pressure-ecmo therapy despite major intracerebral haemorrhage. Anasthesiologie, Intensivmedizin, Notfallmedizin, Schmerztherapie. 2017;**52**:376-381

[35] Faguer S, Saint-Cricq M, Nogier MB, Labadens I, Lavayssiere L, Kamar N, et al. Heparin-free prolonged intermittent hemodialysis using calcium-free citrate dialysate in critically ill patients. Critical Care Medicine. 2017;**45**(11):1887-1892. DOI: 10.1097/CCM.0000000000002694

[36] Shum HP, Kwan AM, Chan KC, Yan WW. The use of regional citrate anticoagulation continuous venovenous hemofiltration in extracorporeal membrane oxygenation. ASAIO Journal. 2014;**60**(4):413-418. DOI: 10.1097/MAT.0000000000000085

[37] Morimont P, Habran S, Desaive T, Blaffart F, Lagny M, Amand T, et al. Extracorporeal CO_2 removal and regional citrate anticoagulation in an experimental model of hypercapnic acidosis. Artificial Organs. 2019;**43**(8): 719-727. DOI: 10.1111/aor.13431

[38] Jibalba J, Sufan JL, Godoy JA. Controversias en la retirada de la ventilación mecánica y extubación en el paciente neurocrítico. Medicina Intensiva. 2018;**42**(9):551-555

[39] Cinotti R, Bouras M, Roquilly A, Asehnoune K. Management and weaning from mechanical ventilation in neurologic patients. Annals of Translational Medicine. 2018;**6**(19):381. DOI: 10.21037/atm.2018.08.16

[40] Boles JM, Bion J, Connors A, Herridge M, et al. European Respiratory Journal. 2007;**29**(5):1033-1056

[41] Fan E, Zakhary B, Amaral A, et al. Liberation from mechanical ventilation in critically Ill adults. An official ATS/ ACCP clinical practice guideline. Annals of the American Thoracic Society. 2017;**14**(3):441-443

[42] Mahanes D, Lewis R. Weaning of the neurologically impaired patient. Critical Care Nursing Clinics of North America. 2004;**16**:387-393

[43] Namen A, Ely E, Tatter S, Case L, Lucia M, Smith A, et al. Predictors of successful extubation in neurosurgical patients. American Journal of Respiratory and Critical Care Medicine. 2001;**163**:658-664

[44] Asehnoune K, Seguin P, Lasocki S, Roquilly A, Delater A, Gros A, et al. Extubation success prediction in a multicentric cohort of patients with severe brain injury. Anesthesiology. 2017;**127**:338-346

[45] Ko R, Ramos L, Chalela J. Conventional weaning parameters do not predict extubation failure in neurocritical care patients. Neurocritical Care. 2009;**10**:269-273

[46] Navalesi P, Frigerio P, Moretti M, Sommariva M, Vesconi S, Baiardi P, et al. Rate of reintubation in mechanically ventilated neurosurgical and neurologic patients: Evaluation of asystematic approach to weaning and extubation.

Critical Care Medicine. 2008; **36**:2986-2992

[47] Manno E, Rabinstein A, Wijdicks E, Brown A, Freeman W, Lee V, et al. A prospective trial of elective extubation in brain injured patients meeting extubation criteria for ventilatory support: A feasibility study. Critical Care. 2008;**12**:R138

[48] Asehnoune K, Roquilly A, Cinotti R. Respiratory management in patients with severe brain injury. Critical Care. 2018;**22**(1):76

[49] Battaglini D, Siwicka Gieroba D, Brunetti I, et al. Mechanical ventilation in neurocritical care setting: A clinical approach. Best Practice & Research. Clinical Anaesthesiology. 2021; **35**(2):207-220

[50] Wang S, Zhang L, Huang K, Lin Z, Qiao W, et al. Predictors of extubation failure in neurocritical patients identified by a systematic review and meta-analysis. PLoS One. 2014;**9**(12): e112198. DOI: 10.1371/journal.pone. 0112198

[51] Coplin W, Pierson D, Cooley K, Newell D, Rubenfeld G. Implications of extubation delay in brain-injured patients meeting standard weaning criteria. American Journal of Respiratory and Critical Care Medicine. 2000;**161**:1530-1536

[52] McCredie V, Ferguson N, Pinto R, Adhikari N, Fowler R, Chap-man M, et al. Airway management strategies for brain-injured patients meeting standard criteria to consider extubation: A prospective cohort study. Annals of the American Thoracic Society. 2017; **14**:85-93

[53] Sarper A, Ayten A, Eser I, Ozbudak O, Demircan A. Tracheal stenosis after tracheostomy or intubation: Review with special regard to cause and management. Texas Heart Institute Journal. 2005;**32**(2):154-158

[54] Quiñones-Ossa GA, Durango-Espinosa YA, Padilla-Zambrano H, et al. Current status of indications, timing, management, complications, and outcomes of tracheostomy in traumatic brain injury patients. Journal of Neurosciences in Rural Practice. 2020;**11**(2):222-229

[55] Andriolo BNG et al. Early versus late tracheostomy for critically ill patients. Cochrane Database of Systematic Reviews. 2015;**1**(1):CD007271

[56] Cheung NH, Napolitano LM. Tracheostomy: Epidemiology, indications, timing, technique, and outcomes. Respiratory Care. 2014; **59**(6):895-915

[57] Dunham CM, Cutrona AF, Gruber BS, Calderon JE, Ransom KJ, Flowers LL. Early tracheostomy in severe traumatic brain injury: Evidence for decreased mechanical ventilation and increased hospital mortality. International Journal of Burns and Trauma. 2014;**4**(1):14-24

[58] Alali AS, Scales DC, Fowler RA, et al. Tracheostomy timing in traumatic brain injury. Journal of Trauma and Acute Care Surgery. 2014;**76**:70-78

[59] McCredie VA et al. Effect of early versus late tracheostomy or prolonged intubation in critically ill patients with acute brain injury: A systematic review and meta-analysis. Neurocritical Care. 2005;**26**(1):14-25

[60] Bösel J, Schiller P, Hook Y, et al. Stroke-related early tracheostomy versus prolonged orotracheal Intubation in neurocritical care trial (SETPOINT): A randomized pilot trial. Stroke. 2013;**44**(1):21-28

[61] Robba C, Galimberti S, Graziano F, et al. Tracheostomy practice and timing in traumatic brain-injured patients: A CENTER-TBI study. Intensive Care Medicine. 2020;**46**:983-994

[62] Schönenberger S, Al-Suwaidan F, Kieser M, Uhlmann L, Bösel J. The SET score to predict tracheostomy need in cerebrovascular neurocritical care patients. Neurocritical Care. 2016;**25**:94-104. DOI: 10.1007/s12028-015-0235-5

[63] Alsherbini K, Goyal N, Metter EJ, et al. Predictors for tracheostomy with external validation of the stroke-related early tracheostomy score (SETscore). Neurocritical Care. 2019;**30**(1):185-192

[64] Johnson-Obaseki S, Veljkovic A, Javidnia H. Complication rates of open surgical versus percutaneous tracheostomy in critically ill patients. Laryngoscope. 2016;**126**(11):2459-2467

[65] Klotz R, Probst P, Deininger M, et al. Percutaneous versus surgical strategy for tracheostomy: A systematic review and meta-analysis of perioperative and postoperative complications. Langenbeck's Archives of Surgery. 2018;**403**(2):137-149

[66] Putensen C, Theuerkauf N, Guenther U, Vargas M, Pelosi P. Percutaneous and surgical tracheostomy in critically ill adult patients: A meta-analysis. Critical Care. 2014;**18**(6):544

Section 3

Weaning and Withdrawal of Mechanical Ventilation

Chapter 6

Weaning from Mechanical Ventilation

Liran Statlender and Pierre Singer

Abstract

Weaning off mechanical ventilation (MV) is a process that ultimately ends with a patient's liberation from the ventilator. As extubation failure worsens prognosis, every effort should be made to safely extubate the patient when the clinical condition allows it. There are several methods and techniques to assess whether a patient is ready for weaning. The clinician should choose the proper method for each patient to minimalize the risk of extubation failure. When liberation from MV is not possible, tracheostomy and transferring the patient to a long-term rehabilitation ward may be required. If this is not feasible, palliative care should be considered.

Keywords: weaning, extubation, spontaneous breathing trial (SBT), rapid shallow breathing index (RSBI)

1. Introduction

Weaning from mechanical ventilation (MV) is the process by which a patient is liberated from a ventilator. It begins with a readiness assessment and ends with liberation, usually by extubation. A successful weaning process should discriminate patients who might fail in the extubation and need reintubation from those who might be successful and maintain spontaneous breathing without mechanical support. This is important, as extubation failure and reintubation worsen prognosis and increase risk of mortality, length of stay, length of ventilation, and ventilation-associated events [1].

Ventilation duration affects the weaning process. If a patient was ventilated for a short time (e.g., during a surgical procedure, trauma patient emergency work-up and treatment), it is usually possible to liberate the patient from MV immediately at the end of the procedure without any special difficulties. Of course, patient characteristics matter in these cases (more caution is mandated in a fragile patient than in a young patient). However, longer time of ventilation due to severe respiratory failure or other severe injury or inflammatory process usually mandates a more structured weaning process, which this chapter describes [2, 3].

2. Readiness for weaning

A daily assessment of readiness for extubation should be performed in every ventilated patient. This screening is important to identify patients who might be successfully weaned and to avoid premature extubation in patients who are not ready yet.

The first consideration when weaning a patient from MV is whether the disease that necessitated MV is controlled and in recovery phase. If the disease process is active and not controlled, the patient should not be considered ready for extubation [4].

The second consideration is respiratory function, both oxygenation and ventilation [5]:

1. Oxygenation

   a. $paO_2/FiO_2 > \sim 260$

   b. $FiO_2 < 0.4$

   c. Positive end expiratory pressure (PEEP) < 5 cmH_2O

If these criteria are not met, it is likely that the patient needs considerable oxygen supplementation.

2. Ventilation

   a. $pH > 7.25$

A lower pH represents a great load on the respiratory system.

These criteria are considered conservative. For example, early works considered paO_2/FiO_2 of 150 as satisfactory for extubation consideration. Later works suggested a higher cutoff of 260–290 [6–8]. Nevertheless, in specific subgroups of patients, these criteria should be slightly adapted. For example, in patients who suffer interstitial lung disease (or other chronic hypoxic diseases), a $paO_2/FiO_2 > 120$ can be used. In patients who suffers from obstructive lung disease, pH and pCO_2 should be close to the patient's baseline level.

The third consideration is cardiovascular function. Initiation of MV unloads the work of breathing from the patient. Cessation of MV imposes this work on the patient again and adds work to the cardiac output. Moreover, as positive end-expiratory pressure (PEEP) decreases afterload, discontinuation of MV increases afterload, potentially worsening heart failure. Therefore, it is necessary that a patient be hemodynamically stable before weaning (no more than a small and stable rate of vasopressors) [9].

The fourth consideration is neurological status. A patient can be considered ready for extubation if they are alert and cooperative. It is necessary that the patient not be under the effect of IV sedation drugs [4], which might cause respiratory depression (opiates, benzodiazepines, propofol). A small dose of IV sedatives that do not cause respiratory depression (dexmedetomidine, ketamine) is acceptable. Enteral or transdermal analgesia and sedation are possible, as long as the doses are stable and the patient is cooperative.

It is worth emphasizing the importance of patient cooperation. After extubation, the patient will usually have to promote cough, cooperate with respiratory therapy, and might need some support in the form of non-invasive ventilation (NIV) or supplementary oxygen. Failure to cooperate with any of these might lead to re-intubation and thus it is important to achieve the patient's cooperation.

Another issue of neurological status is muscle power, especially the ability to cough [10]. Although specific maneuvers to assess respiratory muscle strength are not superior to current maneuvers to assess weaning probability success, it is important to evaluate the patient's ability to cough, as coughing evacuates secretions and prevents aspiration. Whenever a patient seems too weak or not able to perform cough mechanics, the risk of aspiration and re-intubation increases.

Other factors to consider are hemoglobin [11] and temperature [12]. Although both are not mandatory and critical to be completely normal before extubation, it is worth confirming that the patient being assessed for weaning is not developing a new problem such as sepsis, bleeding, or hemolysis (any of which might impose further load on the respiratory system and mandate intubation by itself). If so, it might be better to hold off on the weaning process.

2.1 Weaning predictors

When a patient seems ready for extubation, it is possible to perform some measurements as predictors of successful weaning. As no predictor is 100% sensitive and specific, and as some are cumbersome to perform, it is not mandatory to use any of these predictors. Some use weaning predictors in a structured fashion, while others use them only in cases of doubt whether the patient is ready or not [13–15].

The best studied predictor is the Rapid Shallow Breathing Index (RSBI), which is calculated by dividing the tidal volume (in liters) by the respiratory rate (Vt/f). To calculate this predictor, the patient has to breath spontaneously, without any support, for 1 minute, during which the tidal volume and the respiratory rate are measured. Though this measurement is sometimes performed while disconnecting the patient from the ventilator (measurement by external spirometer), it is acceptable to measure RSBI 1 minute after setting the ventilator on zero pressure support and zero PEEP. An RSBI of 105 is considered the cutoff for extubation failure. RSBI >105 has good correlation with extubation failure (negative predictive value 95%), and thus it is advised to delay extubation. However, RSBI <105 does not guarantee successful weaning, as its positive predictive value is about 80%. Interestingly, using automatic tube compensation increases RSBI sensitivity for successful extubation [13, 16, 17].

Other predictors include p/F ratio, dead space measurement, minute ventilation, compliance of respiratory system, work of breathing, P0.1 (inspiratory effort at 0.1 seconds inspirium), maximal inspiratory pressure (MIP), P0.1/MIP, diaphragmatic sonography, tension-time index (TTI), CROP index, CORE index, Weaning Index (WI), and Integrative Weaning Index (IWI). **Table 1** provides more detail about these predictors [13, 18–24]. Although some of these have been shown to better predict successful or unsuccessful extubation than RSBI, there is only slight improvement in prediction, and all these slightly better predictions are more cumbersome to perform than RSBI.

2.2 Spontaneous breathing trial (SBT)

Whether any weaning predictor is used or not, assessing a patient for extubation requires a spontaneous breathing trial. Several techniques are possible, but the basic principle is the same. The spontaneous breathing trial (SBT) is a short period of time in which the patient is breathing spontaneously, with support as minimal as necessary to overcome the endotracheal tube or without support at all. Among the different techniques are using a T-piece device and ventilating using pressure support mode with pressure support (PS) of 0 cmH_2O and PEEP 0 cmH_2O, or PS 0 cmH_2O and PEEP 5 cmH_2O (CPAP), or PS 7–8 cmH_2O and PEEP 5 cmH_2O. There are controversial results from several studies regarding the superiority of specific techniques. Some studies found no difference, while others have shown better success rates with PSV 8 cmH_2O and PEEP 0 cmH_2O compared to T-piece [25]. In any case, FiO_2 during SBT should be 0.4 or lower.

Predictor name	Description	Successful extubation cutoff	Sens	Spec	PPV	NPV
RSBI	RR/Vt	≤105	0.97	0.64	0.78	0.95
Dead space	$\frac{P_{aCO_2} - P_{eCO_2}}{P_{aCO_2}}$	≥0.58*	0.88	0.85	0.62	0.98
Minute ventilation	RR × Vt	≤15	0.78	0.18	0.55	0.38
Dynamic compliance	$\frac{Vt}{PIP - PEEP}$	≥33	0.72	0.50	0.65	0.58
WOB	Vt × P_{TP}	Not defined				
$P_{0.1}$	Pressure at 0.1 sec during maximal inspiratory effort	≤−4.2	0.87	0.61	0.87	0.61
MIP	Maximal pressure during maximal inspiratory effort	≤−25	0.73	0.28	0.75	0.26
$P_{0.1}$/MIP	$\frac{P_{0.1}}{MIP}$	≤−14	0.98	0.61	0.88	0.92
Diaphragm sonography	Sonographic measurement of diaphragm thickness	<24%	0.93	0.58	0.69	0.89
TTI	$\frac{MAP \times T_i}{MIP \times T_{TOT}}$	≥0.18*	1	1	1	1
CROP	$\frac{C_{DYN} \times MIP \times \frac{P_{aO_2}}{P_{AO_2}}}{RR}$	≥13	0.81	0.57	0.71	0.70
CORE	$\frac{C_{DYN} \times \frac{MIP}{P_{0.1}} \times \frac{P_{aO_2}}{P_{AO_2}}}{RR}$	≥8	1	0.95	0.96	1
IWI	$\frac{C_{RS} \times Sat_{O_2}}{RSBI}$	≥25	0.97	0.94	0.99	0.86

**Dead space and TTI predict failed extubation.*
Sens, sensitivity; Spec, specificity; PPV, positive predictive value; NPV, negative predictive value; RSBI, rapid shallow breathing index; RR, respiratory rate; Vt, tidal volume; P_{aCO_2}, arterial partial pressure of carbon dioxide; P_{eCO_2}, end tidal partial pressure of carbon dioxide; PIP, peak inspiratory pressure; PEEP, positive end expiratory pressure; P_{TP}, transthoracic pressure; MIP, maximal inspiratory pressure; TTI, tension time index; MAP, mean airway pressure; Ti, inspirium time; T_{TOT}, total time of inspirium + expirium; Cdyn, dynamic compliance of lung; P_{aO_2}, arterial pressure of oxygen; P_{AO_2}, alverolar pressure of oxygen; RR, respiratory rate.

Table 1.
Weaning predictors and their diagnostic value.

From a historical point of view, SBT was found to shorten weaning time more than previously used methods of weaning such as PSV gradual decrease, IMV gradual decrease, or no SBT at all [4, 26]. In recent years, an automated mode of SBT has been possible due to the development of closed-loop ventilators. These ventilation modes are mainly pressure controlled/pressure supported, but their settings are changed automatically by the ventilator based on oxygen saturation and end tidal monitoring. Upon activation of automated SBT modes, the ventilator decreases support and monitors physiological parameters including heart rate (from saturation pulse), oxygen saturation, respiratory rate, tidal volume, compliance, end tidal CO_2, and RSBI. After completing SBT for a predefined time, the ventilator alerts whether the patient is ready for extubation or not. There is paucity of data comparing automated SBT to manual SBT, but results seem promising, with a possibility of automated SBT shortening MV duration [27].

When first introduced, the recommendation was to perform SBT for 2 hours. Later studies showed no difference in outcomes with SBT lasting only 30 minutes. When there is a suspicion regarding patient strength, it seems logical to perform longer SBT [28].

As SBT is somewhat challenging for the patient, its endpoint is mainly clinical [5]. To successfully pass the SBT, the patient should remain calm during the test, without any stress signs such as tachycardia, tachypnea, elevated/decreased blood pressure, desaturation, restlessness, feeling uncomfortable, increased effort in breathing, diaphoresis, or new complaints such as chest pain. If any of these occur, the patient has failed the SBT and should remain ventilated. In case of doubt, it is possible to obtain an arterial blood gas (ABG) sample to assess adequacy of oxygenation and ventilation. An ABG sample is also warranted in the case of chronic obstructive pulmonary disease (COPD).

If a patient passes the SBT successfully, extubation should be performed. If a patient fails the SBT, the ventilator should be set to the pre-SBT settings and a workup should be done to determine cause of failure reason and proper treatment. In this case, a daily SBT should take place.

3. Extubation

Once the patient has successfully passed an SBT, extubation should be performed. However, one must pay attention to the patient's ability to remove secretions on their own. Nursing staff should be asked about amounts of secretions and frequency of secretion suctions. Also, patient cough mechanics should be assessed clinically. It is possible that a patient will be screened successfully for extubation and pass an SBT but still suffer from a large amount of secretions or muscle weakness. Suction frequency greater than once every 2 hours is considered unsafe for extubation. Peak expiratory flow during cough <60 L/min is also considered unsafe for extubation. If this is the case, postponing extubation is advised [29].

In select groups of patients who are considered to have risk factors for post-extubation stridor, usually due to laryngeal edema, a cuff leak test is necessary before extubation. This test is not mandatory in all patients, as without any risk factors the leak test is not sensitive nor specific. Risk factors for laryngeal edema include age older than 80 years, female gender, prolonged ventilation (more than 1 week), large-diameter endotracheal tube (more than 8 mm for males and 7 mm for females; smaller diameters are appropriate if the patient is short), CT imaging with endotracheal tube diameter >0.45 than tracheal diameter, Glasgow Coma Scale (GCS) < 8, traumatic intubation, and history of asthma. Any one of these endanger the patient for stridor and therefore mandate performing a cuff leak test. The cuff leak test is performed by deflating the endotracheal tube cuff and measuring the difference between the inspired tidal volume to the expired tidal volume (during volume-controlled ventilation). Generally, when a patient suffers from laryngeal edema, there will be small air leak, if any. Usual cutoffs that support this diagnosis are leak of <110–130 ml or <12–24% of the inhaled tidal volume. If the cuff leak test is positive (i.e., the patient suffers from laryngeal edema), a course of steroids should be given (methylprednisolone 20 mg every 6 hours) before next evaluation [30].

When the patient is ready for extubation, all necessary arrangements should be made to perform the procedure safely. The physician who performs the extubation must keep in mind that despite taking all precautions, the patient might fail immediately and be prepared for reintubation. This is the main theme of the extubation.

Once the decision to extubate the patient is made, FiO_2 of the ventilator should be set to 1. This is the preoxygenation for possible reintubation. All the equipment needed to intubate must be within grasp, including sedation drugs, laryngoscope, endotracheal tube (usually half the size of the current tube), suction tube, and resuscitation cart. If prior intubation of the patient was difficult, then the method that was finally used should be available. Before extubation, a suction is performed within the tube and oral cavity to prevent aspiration. The patient is placed in the upright position and a short explanation about the procedure is given. Extubation itself is performed either with a bag valve mask (e.g., Ambu bag) without one. With an Ambu bag the cuff is deflated, and small positive pressure is constantly applied with the bag while pulling the tube out. Without a bag, the patient is asked to take a deep breath and hold. In that time the cuff is deflated, and the tube is quickly removed. The purpose of both techniques is to set exhalation by the patient as the first movement without the tube to decrease the chance of aspiration.

3.1 Post extubation management

Usually, immediately after extubation the patient is supported by oxygen. Respiratory therapies are advised shortly after the extubation to support secretion removal. Closed monitoring for any sign of respiratory distress is mandatory to allow intervention and reintubation, if necessary, as soon as possible after respiratory distress appears.

About 85% of patients are at low risk of reintubation. Usually, these patients are managed with low-flow oxygen (nasal prongs, simple mask). Occasionally, a patient will be more comfortable with a high-flow nasal canula (HFNC), even without overt hypoxemia. Patients in this group should be monitored closely for 12–24 hours, and if there are no alarming events, they can be discharged from the ICU afterwards (considering no other active ICU problems) [2, 31].

About 15% of patients are at high risk of reintubation within 48 hours of extubation. These patients should be closely monitored and treated accordingly to avoid reintubation. High-risk patients are considered those whose cough is ineffective, who need secretion suction at a frequency greater than one suction every 2 hours, who are in positive fluid balance, who were intubated because of pneumonia. Who are not fully conscious, and who suffer from congestive heart failure (CHF) or COPD. Treatment should be focused with the etiology of deterioration (frequent secretion suction, diuretics, etc.) [1].

Applying HFNC or NIV to these patients seems beneficial in some instances, but this has not been proven. Applying NIV to all extubated patients was not found efficient in all studies performed. In select patients, immediate use of HFNC or NIV might be beneficial, especially in those patients who suffer from COPD or CHF. Both of these patient populations have specific indications for PEEP and therefore have better outcomes when extubated directly to bilevel positive airway pressure (BiPAP). HFNC was found to be non-inferior to NIV, in that instance [32, 33].

When a patient develops respiratory failure after extubation, applying NIV or HFNC might be harmful, as usually it does not prevent reintubation, but rather only postpones it. As such, when the patient finally goes to reintubation, their muscle fatigue is greater than before the NIV/HFNC challenge [4, 34]. Therefore, when a patient starts to deteriorate after extubation, careful monitoring should be performed. If an etiology of deterioration is evident, it must be treated aggressively (suction of secretions, CHF treatment, etc.). If no such reason is apparent, or if treatment response is not sufficient, it is better to reintubate the patient than to challenge with NIV/HFNC.

Reintubation is a bad prognostic factor. Usually, reintubated patients are hospitalized for a longer time (both in ICU and in hospital), suffer from more infections, and have higher mortality rates [1].

4. Management of SBT failure and the difficult-to-wean patient

Approximately 60% of patients manage to pass their first SBT and are extubated successfully. These patients are classified as having simple extubation. About 40% of patients do not pass their first SBT and thus will be classified (initially) as difficult to wean (**Table 2**). These patients should undergo workup to determine why SBT failure occurred. While determining reasons for failure, daily SBT should take place. Most patients who are difficult to wean will require up to three SBTs or 7 days to pass an SBT [2].

Several pathophysiological processes might cause SBT failure. These are classified according to the main system that compromises the patient.

1. Respiratory/ventilatory: hypoxemia, V/Q mismatch, sepsis (excessive CO_2 production), increased airway resistance (COPD/asthma), dynamic hyperinflation, increased secretions, atelectasis, pleural effusion, pneumothorax, ventilator circuit malfunction

2. Cardiac: CHF deterioration, fluid overload

3. Neurological: decreased respiratory drive, oversedation, delirium, anxiety

4. Muscular: respiratory muscle weakness, electrolyte disorders (hypophosphatemia, hypomagnesemia, hypocalcemia, hypokalemia), neuropathy or myopathy, underfeeding, protein catabolism, hypothyroidism

Usually, a careful patient examination involving history review, physical examination, ventilator graph analysis, basic laboratory examination, and imaging studies might reveal the reason and aid treatment.

During the time between SBTs the patient should be ventilated in settings that will maintain oxygenation and ventilation targets, in accordance with lung protective ventilation principles. Usually, PSV mode would apply. However, the patient must be comfortable with PSV settings. In addition, to allow respiratory muscles to rest, some patients may require mandatory ventilation.

Once the process that is suspected to have failed the previous SBT is treated, the patient can undergo another SBT. Usually, this SBT should be longer than the previous one, about 2 hours. The SBT technique should be the same as the previous attempt. However, if CHF is suspected as the reason for SBT failure, it might be better to perform an SBT with a T-piece. This will allow to examine whether the patient can tolerate absence of PEEP.

If the patient successfully passes the SBT, an extubation should be performed. However, if the patient fails, the SBT should be halted at the first signs of failure to decrease fatigue of respiratory muscles.

4.1 Prolonged weaning/prolonged mechanical ventilation

Patients who are not able to pass an SBT in three consecutive attempts or who take more than a week to pass are considered to be going through prolonged weaning. Although they represent the minority (about 10%), these patients are at increased risk of death and are likely to need tracheostomy [3].

Group	Description	Proportion of patients (%)
Simple weaning	Successful extubation at the first attempt of weaning process	85
Difficult weaning	Failure of extubation or SBT at the first attempt, but successful extubation with two further attempts and within 1 week	10–15
Prolonged weaning	At least three failures of extubation or SBTs or duration of weaning process is longer than a week	5

Adapted from Boles et al. [2]

Table 2.
Weaning process classification.

Assuming the acute illness has already recovered, and those pathologies that might cause SBT failure were also treated, the most prominent reason for prolonged MV is imbalance between respiratory system load and capacitance. In other words, patients who need prolonged MV are patients whose respiratory systems cannot meet the physiological demands of the body, whether because of lung pathology (abnormal lung mechanics), respiratory muscle weakness, or neurological dysfunction [31].

Medically, a patient who needs prolonged MV should undergo tracheostomy. This is done to improve patient communication, decrease sedation, ease nursing treatment, and allow for transfer to a long-term weaning facility. With coordination of physicians, nurses, physical therapists, clinical dietitians, and social workers, long-term weaning facilities focus on weaning and rehabilitation. As reasons of prolonged MV are multifactorial, there is no accepted strategy to liberate a patient from the ventilator, and a tailored approach to each patient is feasible.

Outcomes of long-term rehabilitation wards are as follows:

- About 55% of patients are successfully weaned. Average time to wean is approximately 30 days (at the rehabilitation ward). Approximately 40% of these patients survive 1 year.

- About 15% of patients remain ventilator dependent (inability to wean within 3 months). One-year survival in this group is about 20%.

- About 30% of patients die during admission.

One-year survival is variable among different studies, in the range of 25–75%. Most likely, this represents variability in patients' baseline characteristics [35].

Upon diagnosing a patient as one who needs prolonged MV, it is important to discuss this with the patient (or the patient's next of kin/primary caregiver/legal guardian) and explain the chances of remaining ventilator dependent and possible quality of life. If patient expectations are not possible to meet, it seems appropriate to discuss the option of palliative care.

5. Conclusion

Weaning is the process of liberating a patient from MV. Whenever a patient is ventilated for more than 24 hours, the weaning process should be a structured process. **Figure 1** presents the weaning process as performed in our unit. This allows for patient safety and avoids unnecessary extubation failures, which worsen prognosis.

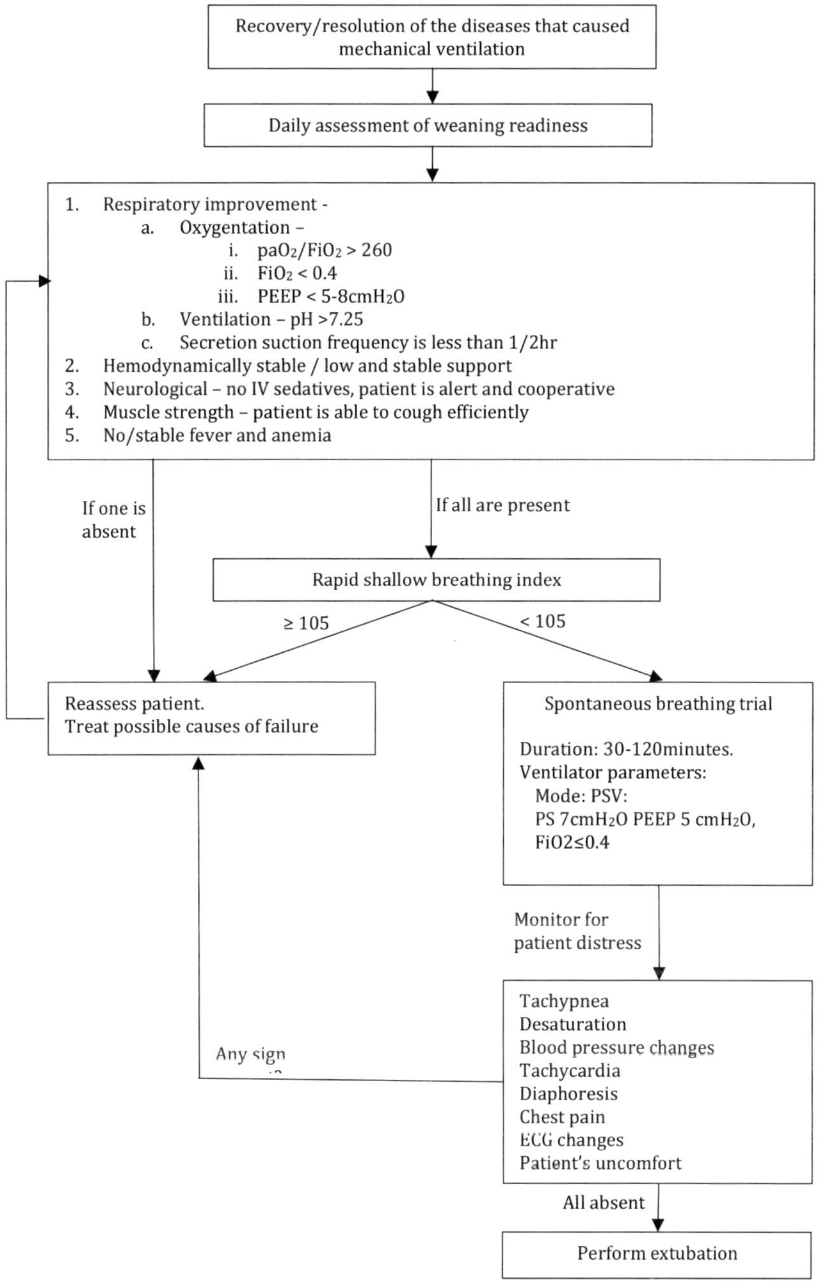

Figure 1.
Suggested flow chart of weaning process.

In most cases, the patient will be extubated without complications. In a minority of cases, special attention should be given to pathological processes that might endanger the patient to extubation failure. In severe cases, weaning will be a long process performed in dedicated ward.

Author details

Liran Statlender* and Pierre Singer
Rabin Medical Center, Petach Tikwa, Israel

*Address all correspondence to: liranst1@clalit.org.il

References

[1] Thille AW, Harrois A, Schortgen F, Brun-Buisson C, Brochard L. Outcomes of extubation failure in medical intensive care unit patients. Critical Care Medicine. 2011;**39**(12):2612-2618

[2] Boles J-M, Bion J, Connors A, Herridge M, Marsh B, Melot C, et al. Weaning from mechanical ventilation. The European Respiratory Journal. 01 May 2007;**29**(5):1033-1056

[3] Peñuelas O, Frutos-Vivar F, Fernández C, Anzueto A, Epstein SK, Apezteguía C, et al. Characteristics and outcomes of ventilated patients according to time to liberation from mechanical ventilation. American Journal of Respiratory and Critical Care Medicine. 15 Aug 2011;**184**(4):430-437

[4] Esteban A, Frutos F, Tobin MJ, Alía I, Solsona JF, Valverdu V, et al. A comparison of four methods of weaning patients from mechanical ventilation. The New England Journal of Medicine. 9 Feb 1995;**332**(6):345-350

[5] MacIntyre NR. Evidence-based guidelines for weaning and discontinuing ventilatory support. Chest. Dec 2001;**120**(6):375S-395S

[6] Wu Y-K, Kao K-C, Hsu K-H, Hsieh M-J, Tsai Y-H. Predictors of successful weaning from prolonged mechanical ventilation in Taiwan. Respiratory Medicine. Aug 2009;**103**(8):1189-1195

[7] Papanikolaou J, Makris D, Saranteas T, Karakitsos D, Zintzaras E, Karabinis A, et al. New insights into weaning from mechanical ventilation: left ventricular diastolic dysfunction is a key player. Intensive Care Medicine. Dec 2011;**37**(12):1976-1985

[8] Savi A, Teixeira C, Silva JM, Borges LG, Pereira PA, Pinto KB, et al. Weaning predictors do not predict extubation failure in simple-to-wean patients. Journal of Critical Care. 2012 Apr;**27**(2):221.e1-221.e8

[9] Richard C, Teboul J-L, Archambaud F, Hebert J-L, Michaut P, Auzepy P. Left ventricular function during weaning of patients with chronic obstructive pulmonary disease. Intensive Care Medicine. Mar 1994;**20**(3):181-186

[10] Salam A, Tilluckdharry L, Amoateng-Adjepong Y, Manthous CA. Neurologic status, cough, secretions and extubation outcomes. Intensive Care Medicine. Jul 2004;**30**(7):1334-1339

[11] Lai Y-C, Ruan S-Y, Huang C-T, Kuo P-H, Yu C-J. Hemoglobin levels and weaning outcome of mechanical ventilation in difficult-to-wean patients: A retrospective cohort study. Rosenberger P, editor. PLoS One. 28 Aug 2013;**8**(8):e73743

[12] Netzer G, Dowdy DW, Harrington T, Chandolu S, Dinglas VD, Shah NG, et al. Fever is associated with delayed ventilator liberation in acute lung injury. Annals of the American Thoracic Society. Dec 2013;**10**(6):608-615

[13] Yang KL, Tobin MJ. A prospective study of indexes predicting the outcome of trials of weaning from mechanical ventilation. The New England Journal of Medicine. 23 May 1991;**324**(21):1445-1450

[14] Conti G, Montini L, Pennisi MA, Cavaliere F, Arcangeli A, Bocci MG, et al. A prospective, blinded evaluation of indexes proposed to predict weaning from mechanical ventilation. Intensive Care Medicine. May 2004;**30**(5):830-836

[15] Epstein SK. Etiology of extubation failure and the predictive value of the rapid shallow breathing index.

American Journal of Respiratory and Critical Care Medicine. Aug 1995;**152**(2):545-549

[16] Desai NR, Myers L, Simeone F. Comparison of 3 different methods used to measure the rapid shallow breathing index. Journal of Critical Care. Aug 2012;**27**(4):418.e1-418.e6

[17] Cohen J, Kogan A, Sahar G, Lev S, Vidne B, Singer P. Hypophosphatemia following open heart surgery: incidence and consequences. European Journal of Cardio-Thoracic Surgery. 1 Aug 2004;**26**(2):306-310

[18] Levy MM, Miyasaki A, Langston D. Work of breathing as a weaning parameter in mechanically ventilated patients. Chest. Oct 1995;**108**(4): 1018-1020

[19] Nemer SN, Barbas CSV, Caldeira JB, Guimarães B, Azeredo LM, Gago R, et al. Evaluation of maximal inspiratory pressure, tracheal airway occlusion pressure, and its ratio in the weaning outcome. Journal of Critical Care. Sep 2009;**24**(3):441-446

[20] Nemer SN, Barbas CS, Caldeira JB, Cárias TC, Santos RG, Almeida LC, et al. A new integrative weaning index of discontinuation from mechanical ventilation. Critical Care. 2009;**13**(5): R152

[21] Harikumar G, Egberongbe Y, Nadel S, Wheatley E, Moxham J, Greenough A, et al. Tension–time index as a predictor of extubation outcome in ventilated children. American Journal of Respiratory and Critical Care Medicine. 15 Nov 2009;**180**(10):982-988

[22] Tenza-Lozano E, Llamas-Alvarez A, Jaimez-Navarro E, Fernández-Sánchez J. Lung and diaphragm ultrasound as predictors of success in weaning from mechanical ventilation. Critical Ultrasound Journal. Dec 2018;**10**(1):12

[23] González-Castro A, Suárez-Lopez V, Gómez-Marcos V, González-Fernandez C, Iglesias-Posadilla D, Burón-Mediavilla J, et al. Valor de la fracción de espacio muerto (Vd/Vt) como predictor de éxito en la extubación. Medicina Intensiva. Dec 2011;**35**(9):529-538

[24] Delisle S, Francoeur M, Albert M, Ouellet P, Bellemare P, Arsenault P. Preliminary evaluation of a new index to predict the outcome of a spontaneous breathing trial. Respiratory Care. 1 Oct 2011;**56**(10):1500-1505

[25] Subirà C, Hernández G, Vázquez A, Rodríguez-García R, González-Castro A, García C, et al. Effect of pressure support vs T-piece ventilation strategies during spontaneous breathing trials on successful extubation among patients receiving mechanical ventilation: A randomized clinical trial. Journal of the American Medical Association. 11 Jun 2019;**321**(22): 2175

[26] Ely EW, Baker AM, Dunagan DP, Burke HL, Smith AC, Kelly PT, et al. Effect on the duration of mechanical ventilation of identifying patients capable of breathing spontaneously. The New England Journal of Medicine. 19 Dec 1996;**335**(25):1864-1869

[27] Burns KE, Lellouche F, Nisenbaum R, Lessard MR, Friedrich JO. Automated weaning and SBT systems versus non-automated weaning strategies for weaning time in invasively ventilated critically ill adults. In: Cochrane Emergency and Critical Care Group, editor. Cochrane Database of Systematic Reviews [Internet]. 2014. Available from: http://doi.wiley.com/10.1002/14651858.CD008638.pub2 [Accessed: 15 June 2021]

[28] Perren A, Domenighetti G, Mauri S, Genini F, Vizzardi N. Protocol-directed weaning from mechanical ventilation: Clinical outcome in patients randomized

for a 30-min or 120-min trial with pressure support ventilation. Intensive Care Medicine. Aug 2002;**28**(8): 1058-1063

[29] Smina M, Salam A, Khamiees M, Gada P, Amoateng-Adjepong Y, Manthous CA. Cough peak flows and extubation outcomes. Chest. Jul 2003;**124**(1):262-268

[30] Jaber S, Chanques G, Matecki S, Ramonatxo M, Vergne C, Souche B, et al. Post-extubation stridor in intensive care unit patients: Risk factors evaluation and importance of the cuff-leak test. Intensive Care Medicine. Jan 2003;**29**(1):69-74

[31] Purro A, Appendini L, De Gaetano A, Gudjonsdottir M, Donner CF, Rossi A. Physiologic determinants of ventilator dependence in long-term mechanically ventilated patients. American Journal of Respiratory and Critical Care Medicine. Apr 2000;**161**(4 Pt 1):1115-1123

[32] Hernández G, Vaquero C, Colinas L, Cuena R, González P, Canabal A, et al. Effect of postextubation high-flow nasal cannula vs noninvasive ventilation on reintubation and postextubation respiratory failure in high-risk patients: A randomized clinical trial. Journal of the American Medical Association. 18 Oct 2016;**316**(15):1565

[33] Nava S, Gregoretti C, Fanfulla F, Squadrone E, Grassi M, Carlucci A, et al. Noninvasive ventilation to prevent respiratory failure after extubation in high-risk patients. Critical Care Medicine. Nov 2005;**33**(11):2465-2470

[34] Keenan SP, Powers C, McCormack DG, Block G. Noninvasive positive-pressure ventilation for postextubation respiratory distress: A randomized controlled trial. Journal of the American Medical Association. 26 Jun 2002;**287**(24):3238

[35] Scheinhorn DJ, Chao DC, Hassenpflug MS, Gracey DR. Post-ICU weaning from mechanical ventilation. Chest. Dec 2001;**120**(6):482S-484S

Chapter 7

How Medical Conditions Affect the Weaning of Mechanical Ventilation

Iuri Christmann Wawrzeniak,
Karolinny Borinelli de Aquino Moura
and Eder Chaves Pacheco

Abstract

Weaning from mechanical ventilation is a common process in critically ill patients and its failure is related to worsening outcomes. A better understanding of the subject is necessary to change these unfavorable results. This chapter will review the approach to weaning from mechanical ventilation in special groups of critically ill patients. The chapter will also review the causes of failure to wean from MV along with strategies for improving evaluation and approach of the patient with difficult and prolonged weaning from mechanical ventilation. Therefore, the presence of this topic in a book on mechanical ventilation is fundamental and relevant.

Keywords: critical illness, intensive care unit, respiratory failure, mechanical ventilation, mechanical ventilator weaning

1. Introduction

Mechanical ventilation (MV) is a lifesaving intervention in critically ill patients. MV is commonly used for postoperative respiratory failure, trauma, pneumonia, sepsis, heart failure (HF), chronic obstructive pulmonary disease (COPD) and acute respiratory distress syndrome (ARDS) [1, 2]. After the condition that caused the use of MV improves, the process of removing invasive ventilatory support begins, which is called weaning from MV [3, 4]. The MV weaning process is crucial and frequent in the critically ill patient's recovery. Almost 50% of the total duration of MV is dedicated to weaning patients [3]. However, some patients may fail to wean from MV despite all criteria in a planned extubation. This extubation failure is reported in around 10–20% of critically ill patients and, consequently, this weaning failure group has a high mortality when compared to patients who successfully weaned from MV [5–9].

The MV weaning and failure process have been studied since the 70s and 80s [10–13]. Milic-Emili questioned that the MV weaning performed in this period was more based on art than science because there were few scientific studies on the topic [14]. Studies in subsequent decades evaluated the best ventilatory mode to perform weaning from MV as well as predictors of weaning from MV [15–19]. After advances in the study of MV weaning, guidelines were formulated establishing better criteria for evaluating the weaning process [20, 21]. Despite this, there are still different ways to practice MV weaning among intensive care units (ICU) in different countries, suggesting the need for more studies on the topic [4].

This chapter aims to review the weaning from MV in special subgroups. How to evaluate and to manage MV weaning will be discussed.

2. Weaning from mechanical ventilation in special groups

The cause of weaning failure may be related to individual or associated dysfunctions (respiratory, muscular, cardiac, neurological, endocrine, metabolic and iatrogenic). However, understanding the pathophysiology of MV weaning failure can be complex in some cases and it is not always fully understood, making its treatment difficult (**Figure 1**). When a patient does not pass a weaning trial, structural evaluation could help to identify factors that played a role in that specific patient. Moreover, it is important to know and to understand peculiarities of some critical patient subgroups in order to achieve more successful weaning. The **Table 1** summarizes the main characteristics, assessment and management of the main groups of patients in the process of weaning from mechanical ventilation admitted to an ICU.

2.1 Chronic obstructive pulmonary disease

In COPD patients, the weaning process is more difficult, prolonged and has higher failure rates than general populations. The higher failure rates in COPD patients can be attributed, at least in part, to the underlying pathophysiology of the disease. In COPD patients with acute respiratory failure, dynamic hyperinflation and the generation of intrinsic PEEP are the main factors that causes increased intrathoracic pressure, which lead to increased work of breathing, MV-induced injury, asynchrony, dyspnea, hemodynamic worsening, in addition to MV dependence and weaning failure [22]. In this population, the use of prophylactic non-invasive ventilation (NIV) after extubation is also recommended, considering this group of patients is at high risk of failure. The use can be extended to immediate extubation for NIV of COPD patients who have failed T-tube spontaneous

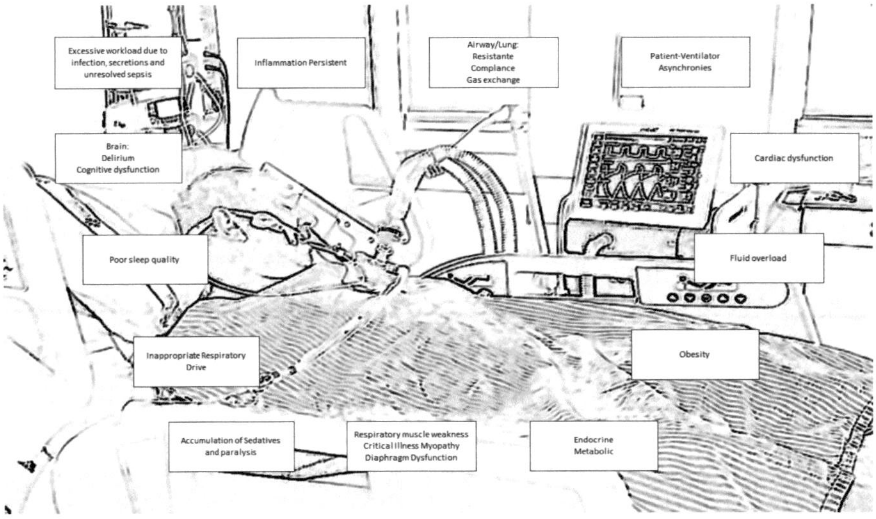

Figure 1.
Aspects of mechanical ventilation weaning failure.

Group	Characteristics	Assessment and Management
COPD	Higher weaning failure and MV dependence Dynamic hyperinflation and intrinsic PEEP	Extubation for NIV
Heart Failure	Increased left ventricular preload which afterload with reduction of the left ventricular ejection fraction	Electrocardiogram and an echocardiography Collecting a pro-brain N-terminal natriuretic peptide/central venous blood gas SvO2 Medications can also be used to optimize ventricular function – inotropic Volume overload should be adjusted - diuretics Extubation for NIV to maintain a PEEP
Neurological Dysfunction	Reduction in the level of consciousness did not impede successful extubation Ability to handle secretions and airway protection are relevant	Daily screening to assess MV weaning CAM-ICU Performing non-pharmacological and pharmacological measures for delirium
Neuromuscular Diseases	Neuromuscular alterations are relatively common Primary neuromuscular disturbance ICU-acquired muscle weakness Diaphragmatic muscle weakness can also impair weaning	Avoiding exposure to medications and hyperglycemia Motor rehabilitation
ARDS	The dangerous of excessive spontaneous ventilation with higher respiratory demands and loss of the protective-ventilation strategy Increased lung volumes, higher respiratory drive, breath stacking, pendelluft and patient-ventilator asynchrony	Evaluation of MV weaning does not differ from others patients Caution in the higher respiratory patients demands and its ventilatory repercussions
Obesity	The large weight on the rib cage can causes alveolar collapse	Higher PEEP during the pre-extubation period to prevent alveolar collapse Use of NIV
Prolonged Weaning	~10% of critically ill intubated patients High mortality Chronic critical illness	Multidisciplinary rehabilitation Swallowing dysfunction Tracheostomy Discussion of treatment goals
Others Care	Conditions for Weaning Progress: • Adequate neurological status • Ability to cough and to manage respiratory secretions • Improvement of oxygenation • Hemodynamic stability	Use of protocols for weaning MV Daily screening for weaning with predictors Use of NIV in ICU patients at high risk for reintubation HFNC reduces the ventilatory work by supplying the demand and reversing the hypoxemic through of a high airflow therapy Cuff Leak Test: high risk of post-extubation stridor (traumatic intubation, prolonged intubation, large endotracheal tube, high cuff pressures, women and reintubation after unplanned extubation) Systemic corticosteroids recommended to patients with fail the cuff leak test Weaning Failure Causes: respiratory, muscular, cardiac, neurological, endocrine, metabolic and iatrogenic

Legend: MV, mechanical ventilation; NIV, non-invasive ventilation; CAM, confusion assessment method; HFNC, High-flow nasal cannula; COPD, chronic obstructive pulmonary disease; PEEP, positive end-expiratory pressure; ARDS, acute respiratory distress syndrome.

Table 1.
Weaning from mechanical ventilation in special groups.

breathing trial (SBT), with evidence of reduced length of stay in the ICU, nosocomial pneumonia and 60-day mortality, when compared to those weaned through invasive pressure support ventilation. These findings were corroborated by a recent meta-analysis [22, 23].

2.2 Heart failure

SBT causes spontaneous respiratory movements, which generate negative pressures and consequently hemodynamic repercussions. Negative intrathoracic pressures cause increased left ventricular (LV) preload which increases LV afterload and, ultimately, reduces left ventricular ejection fraction. This reduction in ejection fraction during an SBT can precipitate or worsen heart failure. Thus, if there are volume overload or systolic or diastolic left ventricular dysfunction, SBT can cause cardiorespiratory decompensation with pulmonary edema, reduced oxygen transport and insufficient cardiac output [24]. Furthermore, SBT can cause or worsen myocardial ischemia as a result of reduced left ventricular compliance, pulmonary edema and/or increased respiratory effort. To assess a possible cardiac dysfunction as a cause of weaning failure, it is suggested to perform an electrocardiogram and an echocardiography, in addition to collecting a pro-brain N-terminal natriuretic peptide and a central venous blood gas measuring SvO2.

An accurate diagnosis of the mechanism of cardiac dysfunction is needed to better guide therapy. In difficult-to-wean patients, additional medications can also be used to optimize ventricular function [24, 25].

Volume overload should be adjusted before performing a SBT because it has been associated with worse weaning outcomes [24]. It can be treated with diuretics or hemodialysis and after that, direct extubation for NIV can be used in order to maintain a positive end-expiratory pressure. When there is evidence of heart pump failure, reduction in afterload and/or use of inotropic agents (such as dobutamine or milrinone) may be considered. Furthermore, the improvement in pulmonary mechanics itself will improve cardiac performance by reducing the afterload of the left ventricle [24].

2.3 Neurological dysfunction

The decision to extubate comatose neurocritical patients is complicated. Previous studies have shown that the reduction in the level of consciousness is a good predictor of extubation failure [26]. Coplin et al. have challenged common sense showing that patients with a Glasgow Coma Scale (GCS) 8 did not impede successful extubation [27]. Moreover, the delayed extubation in this population was related to more ventilator-associated pneumonia (VAP) and longer intensive care unit and hospital stays [28, 29]. Also, according to the study by Coplin et al., the professional should avoid prolonged intubation when the level of consciousness is the only reason to maintain MV. Navalesi et al. demonstrated that a daily screening to assess MV weaning is recommended for patients with neurological diseases to reduce the duration of MV [30]. Strategies that include protective ventilation, early enteral nutrition, standardization of antibiotic therapy for nosocomial pneumonia, and systematic testing to assess readiness for extubation showed an association with a reduction in MV time in brain injured patients [31].

There are still other concerns about the neurological status of patients able to wean from MV. A study has shown that the change in cognitive function had been associated with a four times greater risk of unsuccessful extubation [32]. The ability to handle secretions and airway protection is also a relevant issue. In addition, the causes of acute brain dysfunction in difficult-to-wean patients should be considered, such as delirium, which is very common. The CAM-ICU can be a good tool to assess delirium in intubated ICU patients and performing non-pharmacological and pharmacological measures can help in symptomatic management. Improving hospital environments, for example, with poor noise and ICU-beds near to windows, besides frequent reassurance, touch, verbal orientation and family members presence can improve delirium symptoms [33]. Furthermore, it is important treating potential causal factors such as pain, constipation, infection and withdrawal of precipitating medications such as benzodiazepines and others [25]. In case of hyperactive delirium unresponsive to non-pharmacological measures, antipsychotics can be used for symptomatic management. Although there are no clinically significant differences between the classes of antipsychotics, haloperidol is one of the most used and studied.

2.4 Neuromuscular diseases

Weaning from MV requires adequate neuromuscular activity to overcome the impedance of the respiratory system and maintain adequate alveolar ventilation to eliminate carbon dioxide and ensure a metabolic balance. For this to happen, a generation of the stimulus by the central nervous system, adequate transmission via spinal respiratory motor neurons, respiratory muscles and neuromuscular junctions are necessary. Modifications anywhere of this complex system can contribute to MV weaning failure. Peripheral neurological alterations can also be the cause of weaning failure. Neuromuscular alterations are relatively common, being reported in up to 62% of patients in some studies [34]. Primary neuromuscular disturbance, such as Guillain-Barré syndrome, myasthenia gravis and motor neuron diseases, are usually diagnosed prior to intubation. Occasionally new diagnoses will occur as the difficulty of weaning from MV develops and is investigated.

In the ICU, the most common is secondary neuromuscular diseases, especially muscle weakness acquired in the ICU. It is a pure axonal disease, affecting mainly the peripheral nerves and muscles, symmetrical and bilateral and predominantly proximal. Prevalence between 50 and 100% is estimated in studies and is associated with disease severity, multiorgan dysfunction, exposure to corticosteroids, hyperglycemia and prolonged ICU stay [35–38]. Diaphragmatic muscle weakness can also impair weaning and its assessment can be challenging at the bedside, as the tests are either invasive and/or depend on the patient's ability to understand and to cooperate. There are studies that demonstrate an association between ICU-acquired muscle weakness and longer weaning duration or failure [34, 39–41]. Diaphragmatic muscle weakness can also impair weaning and its assessment can be challenging at the bedside, as the tests are either invasive and/or depend on the patient's ability to understand and to cooperate. There are studies that demonstrate an association between ICU-acquired muscle weakness and longer weaning duration or failure.

2.5 ARDS

In the early stages of MV in patients with acute respiratory distress syndrome (ARDS), the use of protective-ventilation strategies is recommended, as well as the use of neuromuscular blockers, prone position and extracorporeal membrane oxygenation (ECMO) in more severe cases [42]. However, during weaning from MV in patients with ARDS, this protective-ventilation strategy may be lost, mainly due to the influence of spontaneous ventilation with higher respiratory demands [43]. The increased lung volumes, higher respiratory drive, breath stacking, pendelluft and patient-ventilator asynchrony besides to delirium and ICU-acquired paresis may influence weaning from MV and should be considered in the assessment of patients with ARDS [44].

In addition, the use of the arterial-to-inspired oxygen (PaO2/FiO2) ratio to demonstrate improvement in hypoxemia, does not always translate into improvement in inflammatory response and weaning success [45]. Then, the premise for the beginning of weaning from MV based on PaO2/FiO2 ratio (resolution or improvement of the cause that led the patient to MV) is not always a good predictor to weaning success. Moreover, the management of MV weaning in these patients through consensus on weaning from MV generally does not include this specific group of patients [20, 21, 46]. Studies have shown that a greater proportion of patients have difficult and prolonged weaning when compared to the general ICU population [29, 47]. Therefore, regarding current knowledge, the evaluation of MV weaning does not differ in general from other patients. However, this subgroup has a particular pathophysiology that can influence and delay the evolution of the withdrawal of invasive ventilatory support.

2.6 Obesity

Obese patients, with a body mass index (BMI) > 30, have specific problems during MV. The large weight on the rib cage can cause alveolar collapse in some conditions and gravity can influence pulmonary mechanics [48]. In a study of obese patients with ARF, mortality was reduced by 50% when the choice of PEEP was guided with an esophageal catheter (EsoC) and electrical impedance tomography (EIT) [49]. During the process of weaning of MV is crucial to pay attention to the work of breathing, because the increased negative pleural pressure in these patients can led to a compression of the diaphragm in to the rib cage and can induce atelectasis in patients with muscle weakness [49]. Therefore, obese patients may benefit from higher PEEP during the pre-extubation period, making pleural pressure more positive and preventing alveolar collapse [50]. After extubation, positive pressure in the smaller airways can be maintained through by NIV, preferably in a sitting position, to avoid abdominal cavity compression of the diaphragm and inducing collapse by undermining the mechanics of the rib cage [51].

3. Prolonged weaning and some considerations

Prolonged weaning concerns about 10% of critically ill intubated patients and is associated with a high mortality [19, 27, 52]. Patients with prolonged weaning are associated with chronic critical illness [53]. The multidisciplinary rehabilitation group is very important to treatment [54]. Physical therapy will be very important to assess the patient's tolerance and exercise. Swallowing dysfunction can complicate the extubation process and its evaluation is essential for the return to normal eating habits [55]. Short daily cuff down trials with a speaking valve are performed to induce vocal cords to exert their original function during expiration. Tracheostomy may be considered as a useful adjunct for easier care of the patient, especially for mobilization and better comfort [56, 57]. A randomized controlled trial suggested that tracheostomized patients were more rapidly separated from the ventilator by repetitive T-tube trials than with a gradual reduction of PSV without influencing survival at 12 months [58]. Assessment with the patient and family should address explicit discussion of realistic versus futile treatment goals [59].

4. Future perspectives

More recently, tools such as ultrasound, EsoC and EIT have helped to predict MV weaning. The EsoC can be useful in the objective assessment of respiratory effort, estimating transpulmonary pressure and autoPEEP [60]. On the other hand, ultrasound can be useful in providing information through visual assessment and in obtaining objective measurements of cardiorespiratory variables at different stages of weaning. A study by Haji et al. showed that loss of pulmonary aeration and left ventricular diastolic dysfunction are more frequent in patients who fail extubation [61]. Additionally, several studies have shown that the use of the EIT can help to evaluate weaning from MV. Bickenbach et al. and Lima et al. showed loss of recruitment and lung homogeneity during SBT [62, 63]. Studies in specific populations, such as patients with COPD, are ongoing and partial results indicate that those who fail the SBT ventilate more the anterior lung regions [64].

5. Conclusions

The weaning from MV in critically ill patients is a common and fundamental process in the ICU. The understanding the withdrawal of invasive ventilatory support and identifying possible causes of weaning failure are essential. The use of SBT trial and predictors guide weaning from MV. Some subgroups should be better valued to better individualize MV weaning and avoid reintubation associated with worse outcomes.

Conflict of interest

"The authors declare no conflict of interest."

Author details

Iuri Christmann Wawrzeniak[1*], Karolinny Borinelli de Aquino Moura[1,2] and Eder Chaves Pacheco[3]

1 Centro de Terapia Intensiva do Hospital de Clínicas de Porto Alegre, Brazil

2 Programa de Pós-Graduação em Cardiologia da Universidade Federal do Rio Grande do Sul, Brazil

3 Laboratório de Pneumologia LIM-09, Hospital das Clínicas da Faculdade de Medicina, Universidade de São Paulo, Brazil

*Address all correspondence to: iwawrzeniak@hcpa.edu.br

References

[1] Wunsch H, Linde-Zwirble WT, Angus DC, Hartman ME, Milbrandt EB, Kahn JM. The epidemiology of mechanical ventilation use in the United States. Critical care medicine. 2010; 38(10):1947-1953.

[2] Esteban A, Anzueto A, Frutos F, Alia I, Brochard L, Stewart TE, et al. Characteristics and outcomes in adult patients receiving mechanical ventilation: a 28-day international study. Jama. 2002;287(3):345-355.

[3] McConville JF, Kress JP. Weaning patients from the ventilator. The New England journal of medicine. 2012;367(23):2233-2239.

[4] Burns KEA, Raptis S, Nisenbaum R, Rizvi L, Jones A, Bakshi J, et al. International Practice Variation in Weaning Critically Ill Adults from Invasive Mechanical Ventilation. Annals of the American Thoracic Society. 2018;15(4):494-502.

[5] Frutos-Vivar F, Esteban A, Apezteguia C, Gonzalez M, Arabi Y, Restrepo MI, et al. Outcome of reintubated patients after scheduled extubation. Journal of critical care. 2011;26(5):502-509.

[6] Epstein SK, Ciubotaru RL, Wong JB. Effect of failed extubation on the outcome of mechanical ventilation. Chest. 1997;112(1):186-192.

[7] Esteban A, Frutos-Vivar F, Ferguson ND, Arabi Y, Apezteguia C, Gonzalez M, et al. Noninvasive positive-pressure ventilation for respiratory failure after extubation. The New England journal of medicine. 2004;350(24):2452-2460.

[8] Seymour CW, Martinez A, Christie JD, Fuchs BD. The outcome of extubation failure in a community hospital intensive care unit: a cohort study. Critical care. 2004;8(5): R322-R327.

[9] Torres A, Gatell JM, Aznar E, el-Ebiary M, Puig de la Bellacasa J, Gonzalez J, et al. Re-intubation increases the risk of nosocomial pneumonia in patients needing mechanical ventilation. American journal of respiratory and critical care medicine. 1995;152(1):137-141.

[10] Sahn SA, Lakshminarayan S, Petty TL. Weaning from mechanical ventilation. Jama. 1976;235(20): 2208-2212.

[11] Kimball WR, Leith DE, Robins AG. Dynamic hyperinflation and ventilator dependence in chronic obstructive pulmonary disease. The American review of respiratory disease. 1982; 126(6):991-995.

[12] Tobin MJ, Perez W, Guenther SM, Semmes BJ, Mador MJ, Allen SJ, et al. The pattern of breathing during successful and unsuccessful trials of weaning from mechanical ventilation. The American review of respiratory disease. 1986;134(6):1111-1118.

[13] Jubran A, Tobin MJ. Pathophysiologic basis of acute respiratory distress in patients who fail a trial of weaning from mechanical ventilation. American journal of respiratory and critical care medicine. 1997;155(3):906-915.

[14] Milic-Emili J. Is weaning an art or a science? The American review of respiratory disease. 1986;134(6): 1107-1108.

[15] Tomlinson JR, Miller KS, Lorch DG, Smith L, Reines HD, Sahn SA. A prospective comparison of IMV and T-piece weaning from mechanical ventilation. Chest. 1989;96(2):348-352.

[16] Esen F, Denkel T, Telci L, Kesecioglu J, Tutuncu AS, Akpir K, et al. Comparison of pressure support ventilation (PSV) and intermittent mandatory ventilation (IMV) during weaning in patients with acute respiratory failure. Advances in experimental medicine and biology. 1992;317:371-376.

[17] Brochard L, Rauss A, Benito S, Conti G, Mancebo J, Rekik N, et al. Comparison of three methods of gradual withdrawal from ventilatory support during weaning from mechanical ventilation. American journal of respiratory and critical care medicine. 1994;150(4):896-903.

[18] Esteban A, Frutos F, Tobin MJ, Alia I, Solsona JF, Valverdu I, et al. A comparison of four methods of weaning patients from mechanical ventilation. Spanish Lung Failure Collaborative Group. The New England journal of medicine. 1995;332(6):345-350.

[19] Sellares J, Ferrer M, Torres A. Predictors of weaning after acute respiratory failure. Minerva anestesiologica. 2012;78(9):1046-1053.

[20] MacIntyre NR, Cook DJ, Ely EW, Jr., Epstein SK, Fink JB, Heffner JE, et al. Evidence-based guidelines for weaning and discontinuing ventilatory support: a collective task force facilitated by the American College of Chest Physicians; the American Association for Respiratory Care; and the American College of Critical Care Medicine. Chest. 2001;120(6 Suppl):375S-395S.

[21] Schmidt GA, Girard TD, Kress JP, Morris PE, Ouellette DR, Alhazzani W, et al. Official Executive Summary of an American Thoracic Society/American College of Chest Physicians Clinical Practice Guideline: Liberation from Mechanical Ventilation in Critically Ill Adults. American journal of respiratory and critical care medicine. 2017;195(1): 115-119.

[22] Burns KE, Meade MO, Premji A, Adhikari NK. Noninvasive ventilation as a weaning strategy for mechanical ventilation in adults with respiratory failure: a Cochrane systematic review. CMAJ : Canadian Medical Association journal = journal de l'Association medicale canadienne. 2014;186(3): E112-22.

[23] Nava S, Ambrosino N, Clini E, Prato M, Orlando G, Vitacca M, et al. Noninvasive mechanical ventilation in the weaning of patients with respiratory failure due to chronic obstructive pulmonary disease. A randomized, controlled trial. Annals of internal medicine. 1998;128(9):721-728.

[24] Perren A, Brochard L. Managing the apparent and hidden difficulties of weaning from mechanical ventilation. Intensive care medicine. 2013;39(11): 1885-1895.

[25] Heunks LM, van der Hoeven JG. Clinical review: the ABC of weaning failure--a structured approach. Critical care. 2010;14(6):245.

[26] Namen AM, Ely EW, Tatter SB, Case LD, Lucia MA, Smith A, et al. Predictors of successful extubation in neurosurgical patients. American journal of respiratory and critical care medicine. 2001;163(3 Pt 1):658-664.

[27] Coplin WM, Pierson DJ, Cooley KD, Newell DW, Rubenfeld GD. Implications of extubation delay in brain-injured patients meeting standard weaning criteria. American journal of respiratory and critical care medicine. 2000;161(5): 1530-1536.

[28] Thille AW, Cortes-Puch I, Esteban A. Weaning from the ventilator and extubation in ICU. Current opinion in critical care. 2013;19(1):57-64.

[29] Penuelas O, Frutos-Vivar F, Fernandez C, Anzueto A, Epstein SK, Apezteguia C, et al. Characteristics and

outcomes of ventilated patients according to time to liberation from mechanical ventilation. American journal of respiratory and critical care medicine. 2011;184(4):430-437.

[30] Navalesi P, Frigerio P, Moretti MP, Sommariva M, Vesconi S, Baiardi P, et al. Rate of reintubation in mechanically ventilated neurosurgical and neurologic patients: evaluation of a systematic approach to weaning and extubation. Critical care medicine. 2008;36(11): 2986-2992.

[31] Roquilly A, Cinotti R, Jaber S, Vourc'h M, Pengam F, Mahe PJ, et al. Implementation of an evidence-based extubation readiness bundle in 499 brain-injured patients. a before-after evaluation of a quality improvement project. American journal of respiratory and critical care medicine. 2013;188(8): 958-966.

[32] Salam A, Tilluckdharry L, Amoateng-Adjepong Y, Manthous CA. Neurologic status, cough, secretions and extubation outcomes. Intensive care medicine. 2004;30(7):1334-1339.

[33] Landefeld CS, Palmer RM, Kresevic DM, Fortinsky RH, Kowal J. A randomized trial of care in a hospital medical unit especially designed to improve the functional outcomes of acutely ill older patients. The New England journal of medicine. 1995;332(20):1338-1344.

[34] De Jonghe B, Bastuji-Garin S, Sharshar T, Outin H, Brochard L. Does ICU-acquired paresis lengthen weaning from mechanical ventilation? Intensive care medicine. 2004;30(6):1117-1121.

[35] Witt NJ, Zochodne DW, Bolton CF, Grand'Maison F, Wells G, Young GB, et al. Peripheral nerve function in sepsis and multiple organ failure. Chest. 1991;99(1):176-184.

[36] Garnacho-Montero J, Madrazo-Osuna J, Garcia-Garmendia JL, Ortiz-Leyba C, Jimenez-Jimenez FJ, Barrero-Almodovar A, et al. Critical illness polyneuropathy: risk factors and clinical consequences. A cohort study in septic patients. Intensive care medicine. 2001;27(8):1288-1296.

[37] Bercker S, Weber-Carstens S, Deja M, Grimm C, Wolf S, Behse F, et al. Critical illness polyneuropathy and myopathy in patients with acute respiratory distress syndrome. Critical care medicine. 2005;33(4):711-715.

[38] De Jonghe B, Sharshar T, Lefaucheur JP, Authier FJ, Durand-Zaleski I, Boussarsar M, et al. Paresis acquired in the intensive care unit: a prospective multicenter study. Jama. 2002;288(22):2859-2867.

[39] Leijten FS, De Weerd AW, Poortvliet DC, De Ridder VA, Ulrich C, Harink-De Weerd JE. Critical illness polyneuropathy in multiple organ dysfunction syndrome and weaning from the ventilator. Intensive care medicine. 1996;22(9):856-861.

[40] Druschky A, Herkert M, Radespiel-Troger M, Druschky K, Hund E, Becker CM, et al. Critical illness polyneuropathy: clinical findings and cell culture assay of neurotoxicity assessed by a prospective study. Intensive care medicine. 2001;27(4): 686-693.

[41] Garnacho-Montero J, Amaya-Villar R, Garcia-Garmendia JL, Madrazo-Osuna J, Ortiz-Leyba C. Effect of critical illness polyneuropathy on the withdrawal from mechanical ventilation and the length of stay in septic patients. Critical care medicine. 2005;33(2): 349-354.

[42] Papazian L, Aubron C, Brochard L, Chiche JD, Combes A, Dreyfuss D, et al. Formal guidelines: management of acute respiratory distress syndrome. Annals of intensive care. 2019;9(1):69.

[43] Wawrzeniak IC, Regina Rios Vieira S, Almeida Victorino J. Weaning from Mechanical Ventilation in ARDS: Aspects to Think about for Better Understanding, Evaluation, and Management. BioMed research international. 2018;2018:5423639.

[44] Yoshida T, Fujino Y, Amato MB, Kavanagh BP. Fifty Years of Research in ARDS. Spontaneous Breathing during Mechanical Ventilation. Risks, Mechanisms, and Management. American journal of respiratory and critical care medicine. 2017;195(8): 985-992.

[45] Spinelli E, Mauri T. Why improved PF ratio should not be our target when treating ARDS. Minerva anestesiologica. 2021;87(7):752-754.

[46] Boles JM, Bion J, Connors A, Herridge M, Marsh B, Melot C, et al. Weaning from mechanical ventilation. The European respiratory journal. 2007;29(5):1033-1056.

[47] Jeong BH, Ko MG, Nam J, Yoo H, Chung CR, Suh GY, et al. Differences in clinical outcomes according to weaning classifications in medical intensive care units. PloS one. 2015;10(4):e0122810.

[48] Kacmarek RM, Wanderley HV, Villar J, Berra L. Weaning patients with obesity from ventilatory support. Current opinion in critical care. 2021;27(3):311-319.

[49] Obi ON, Mazer M, Bangley C, Kassabo Z, Saadah K, Trainor W, et al. Obesity and Weaning from Mechanical Ventilation-An Exploratory Study. Clinical medicine insights Circulatory, respiratory and pulmonary medicine. 2018;12:1179548418801004.

[50] Teggia Droghi M, De Santis Santiago RR, Pinciroli R, Marrazzo F, Bittner EA, Amato MBP, et al. High Positive End-Expiratory Pressure Allows Extubation of an Obese Patient. American journal of respiratory and critical care medicine. 2018;198(4): 524-525.

[51] Grassi L, Kacmarek R, Berra L. Ventilatory Mechanics in the Patient with Obesity. Anesthesiology. 2020;132(5):1246-1256.

[52] Funk GC, Anders S, Breyer MK, Burghuber OC, Edelmann G, Heindl W, et al. Incidence and outcome of weaning from mechanical ventilation according to new categories. The European respiratory journal. 2010;35(1):88-94.

[53] Macintyre NR. Chronic critical illness: the growing challenge to health care. Respiratory care. 2012;57(6): 1021-1027.

[54] Mauri T, Pivi S, Bigatello LM. Prolonged mechanical ventilation after critical illness. Minerva anestesiologica. 2008;74(6):297-301.

[55] Ceriana P, Carlucci A, Navalesi P, Rampulla C, Delmastro M, Piaggi G, et al. Weaning from tracheotomy in long-term mechanically ventilated patients: feasibility of a decisional flowchart and clinical outcome. Intensive care medicine. 2003;29(5): 845-848.

[56] Rumbak MJ, Newton M, Truncale T, Schwartz SW, Adams JW, Hazard PB. A prospective, randomized, study comparing early percutaneous dilational tracheotomy to prolonged translaryngeal intubation (delayed tracheotomy) in critically ill medical patients. Critical care medicine. 2004;32(8):1689-1694.

[57] Trouillet JL, Luyt CE, Guiguet M, Ouattara A, Vaissier E, Makri R, et al. Early percutaneous tracheotomy versus prolonged intubation of mechanically ventilated patients after cardiac surgery: a randomized trial. Annals of internal medicine. 2011;154(6):373-383.

[58] Jubran A, Grant BJ, Duffner LA, Collins EG, Lanuza DM, Hoffman LA, et al. Effect of pressure support vs unassisted breathing through a tracheostomy collar on weaning duration in patients requiring prolonged mechanical ventilation: a randomized trial. Jama. 2013;309(7):671-677.

[59] Aghabarary M, Dehghan Nayeri N. Medical futility and its challenges: a review study. Journal of medical ethics and history of medicine. 2016;9:11.

[60] Yoshida T, Brochard L. Ten tips to facilitate understanding and clinical use of esophageal pressure manometry. Intensive care medicine. 2018;44(2): 220-2.

[61] Haji K, Haji D, Canty DJ, Royse AG, Green C, Royse CF. The impact of heart, lung and diaphragmatic ultrasound on prediction of failed extubation from mechanical ventilation in critically ill patients: a prospective observational pilot study. Critical ultrasound journal. 2018;10(1):13.

[62] Bickenbach J, Czaplik M, Polier M, Marx G, Marx N, Dreher M. Electrical impedance tomography for predicting failure of spontaneous breathing trials in patients with prolonged weaning. Critical care. 2017;21(1):177.

[63] Lima JNG, Fontes MS, Szmuszkowicz T, Isola AM, Maciel AT. Electrical impedance tomography monitoring during spontaneous breathing trial: Physiological description and potential clinical utility. Acta anaesthesiologica Scandinavica. 2019;63(8):1019-1027.

[64] Moura KBA, Bertoldi RA, Wawrzeniak IC, Balzan F, Pellegrini JAS, Pacheco E, et al. Use of Electrical Impedance Tomography and Esophageal Catheter for Weaning from Mechanical Ventilation of Patients with COPD - A Pilot Study. American journal of respiratory and critical care medicine. 2020;201(A5215).

Chapter 8

Palliative Withdrawal of Mechanical Ventilation and Other Life Supports

Lauren F. Goodman

Abstract

Palliative or compassionate withdrawal of mechanical ventilator support at the end of life aims to optimize comfort, alleviate suffering, and allow a natural death in patients for whom life supports are not achieving desired goals. Palliative withdrawal is a medical procedure and must be treated as such. Appropriate planning and preparations are required to optimize patient comfort, which is the goal of the procedure. Many institutions have a "one size fits all" approach to this process, but individual patient factors require consideration to meet the patient's needs. Some of these factors include patient pathophysiology (airway edema, airway trauma, hemoptysis, secretions), current treatment modalities (ventilator settings, medications including sedatives, vasopressors, inotropes, inhaled agents, neuromuscular blockade agents), and patient and family values and preferences. This chapter will discuss the implications of each of these factors and propose methods for successful transitions to comfort-focused care. Case vignettes will demonstrate the thought processes involved and model optimal management. Common ethical considerations and questions regarding palliative withdrawal of life support will also be discussed.

Keywords: Palliative, terminal, Withdrawal, comfort care, end of life

1. Introduction

Palliative or compassionate withdrawal of mechanical ventilator support at the end of life aims to optimize comfort, alleviate suffering, and allow a natural death in patients for whom life supports are not achieving desired goals. Medical ethics discussions have shifted significantly over the decades since critical care was first developed. It is now generally, though not universally, accepted that withdrawal of life support is equivalent to withholding of life support. Some now argue that withdrawal may be ethically superior to withholding life support, as withholding assumes the life support will not achieve the patient's goal, while withdrawal occurs only after this assumption has been proven true [1].

2. Decision-making process

A patient with capacity must be given the opportunity to participate in decision-making. This can be challenging when medical interventions limit audible speech, as with an oroendotracheal or nasoendotracheal tube. While sometimes time-consuming, solutions such as computers or tablets with keyboards, phones with texting capabilities, sign language, letter boards, or simply pen and paper, can allow a patient to ask questions and express their own values, goals, and preferences. Some patients with a tracheostomy tube in place can generate audible fricative speech, even when the cuff must remain inflated for respiratory support. Some patients with either tube can mouth words clearly enough to be understood, though this can be difficult for both patient and medical team. The powers of the Power of Attorney may be limited by the patient, or by local laws, but generally allow the surrogate to make medical decisions on the patient's behalf when the patient is unable or chooses to defer. Capacity for medical decision-making is a complex construct and can vary over time, and with the decision to be made. Some patients are unable to process any significant medical information. Some are able to process and express clear and consistent preferences about simpler matters but not complex ones. As with language interpretation, these interpretations must be made by a member of the medical team and not exclusively by family or friends of the patient, and must be confirmed with the patient in other ways, such as nodding or shaking their head to confirm or refute accuracy.

A patient with capacity can also choose to defer to their legal surrogate, and in many jurisdictions can select and assign Power of Attorney for Health Care to one or more people to speak for them.

Still others are able to understand, manipulate, and ask questions about the medical information presented to them, and to express clear, consistent decisions on their own behalf.

3. When to discuss withdrawal of life supports

Ideally, physicians discuss with each patient their prior experiences, values, preferences, goals, and minimal acceptable outcomes prior to onset of critical illness, and prior to initiation of life supports. This is often not possible, sometimes due to the acute nature of some critical illnesses, and sometimes due to patient factors such as unwillingness to discuss these issues. Unfortunately, this is also sometimes due to physicians' and medical teams' discomfort with, inadequate time for, or failure to recognize the necessity of such discussions.

Regardless of whether routine or baseline discussions of experiences, values, preferences, and goals have occurred, the onset of critical illness is an important prompt to discuss or rediscuss these thoughts. Ideally, at the beginning of a patient's critical illness, their physician discusses with the patient or surrogate, or with both, the presumed diagnosis, the treatment options, and the likely outcomes of each and how soon the outcomes are anticipated. The patient or surrogate ideally understands and integrates this information and selects the treatment that gives them the best chance of recovery within the parameters of acceptable risk and acceptable burdens or suffering defined by that individual patient. After learning the patient's risk and burden tolerance, the physician confirms and documents the treatment plan, including any limits set by agreement with the patient or surrogate. The physician should then schedule a date to discuss progress, or lack of improvement, and further options with the patient or surrogate, unless new findings or changes require significant discussions sooner. This constitutes a time-limited trial, which is a useful framework for acknowledging the uncertainty of outcomes of critical illness [2].

If the patient is not improving to the extent they themselves would require to make continuing current life supports acceptable, or if the patient, or surrogate acting in the patient's best interest, finds the current life supports too burdensome despite good efforts at symptom management by the medical team, it is important to discuss the option of palliative withdrawal of life supports.

When multiple life supports are present, and the patient or surrogate and team are considering withdrawing one form of life support, it is necessary to consider whether or not the other forms of life support present are contributing to achievable medical goals. If any form of life support is not helping the patient progress toward achievable goals, potential withdrawal should be considered and discussed.

4. How to withdraw mechanical ventilation

Palliative withdrawal is a medical procedure and must be treated as such. Appropriate planning and preparations are required to optimize patient comfort, which is the goal of the procedure. Many previously published works, and many institutions have a "one size fits all" approach to this process, but individual patient factors require consideration to meet the patient's needs. Unfortunately, for understandable reasons, at this time there are exceedingly few studies of how to perform any part of this procedure. Therefore, many aspects require logical consideration and expert opinion to guide practice, as well as consideration of the individual patient's condition, needs, preferences, and goals.

Evidence suggests family satisfaction is increased when a step-wise approach to withdrawal of life support is used [3].

4.1 Ventilator weaning vs. immediate discontinuation

Older literature regarding palliative withdrawal of life supports generally describes either universal weaning or universal immediate discontinuation. More recent literature and guidelines take a more patient-centered, case-specific approach and recommend consideration of the patient's current ventilator support requirements and level of symptoms [4]. For patients on moderate or high ventilator support, it is recommended to wean ventilator support - specifically positive end inspiratory pressure (PEEP), potentially pressure support, and fraction of inspired oxygen (FiO2) - in a step-wise approach, titrating opioids and benzodiazepines especially to control dyspnea and anxiety respectively.

For example, for a patient who is on assist control volume control with a set rate of 14, tidal volume 6 mL/kg ideal body weight, PEEP of 14 cmH2O, and FiO2 60%, it would be advisable to achieve comfort with medications before initiating weaning, then reduce PEEP and FIO2 to 10–12 and 40% respectively, titrate medication boluses to achieve and maintain comfort, and continue to wean ventilator support every 15-30 minutes as tolerated.

4.1.1 Mode

Modern ventilators allow for a wide variety of mandatory, intermittent mandatory, assisted breath, and entirely spontaneous modes. Each mode has potential benefits and potential burdens to the patient.

When transitioning to comfort measures, patient condition and clinician comfort with managing the various modes will determine optimal mode for weaning or continued support. A patient who is awake, alert, and requires little ventilator support may be most comfortable right away with low levels of pressure support and PEEP. A patient with poor lung compliance or with neurologic or myopathic limitations to breathing may require a more sensitive trigger or a more controlled mode that ensures volume delivery, and for some, having a minimum breath frequency is necessary for comfort.

4.1.2 Rate

In modes with a set minimum rate, reducing a rapid set rate may unmask intrinsic tachypnea, which may be physiologic, or may be due to pain or anxiety. In synchronized intermittent mandatory ventilation settings, reducing the set rate may increase the frequency of spontaneous breaths; depending on the level of support provided with these spontaneous breaths, patients may feel more dyspnea if under-supported, or less dyspnea if their respiratory efforts are sufficiently supported.

4.1.3 Peep

Reducing PEEP can allow pulmonary edema, alveolar secretions, or pulmonary hemorrhage to become more prominent. Some patients may experience increased cough and may have difficulty expectorating the secretions. A stepwise approach, reducing PEEP by 2–4 cmH2O per step, may allow for titration of symptom control medications. Most ventilators have backup apnea settings that cannot be discontinued. For patients who are maintained on ventilator support throughout the comfort care process, it is important to remind families and team members that the ventilator will continue to deliver breaths even after the patient has died.

4.1.4 Oxygen

Some patients are asymptomatic or relatively asymptomatic with hypoxemia, while others note symptoms with even relatively small reductions in oxygenation. Again a stepwise approach, reducing by approximately 20% per step, allows for symptom management with medication titration. Supplemental oxygen through the ventilator can be weaned to as low as 21%, especially if the plan is for discontinuation of ventilator support without supplemental oxygen.

4.1.5 Tidal volume

Since the first ARDSnet trial publication [5], when tidal volumes are set on the ventilator, they are commonly set to a low tidal volume, lung protective strategy of 8 mL or less per kilogram of ideal body weight. Some patients find this strategy uncomfortable, as it forces small, limited volume breaths. If ventilator support is to be continued, especially if awaiting arrival of family members, or another significant event, continuing the current set volume is typical, but liberalizing the set volume somewhat may improve comfort.

4.1.6 Drive pressure, inspiratory pressure, or pressure support

These terms all refer to pressure added by the ventilator for the inspiratory phase of each breath to inflate the lungs and generate a tidal volume. The size of the tidal volume depends on the pressure administered and on the patient's lung and airway compliance. For patients with acute lung injury or acute respiratory distress syndrome, the pressure is generally set to target lung protective low tidal volumes. For patients without lung injury, the pressure requirement may be fairly low, or may be set to allow more liberal breath sizes for comfort.

4.2 Extubating vs. maintaining oro- or nasoendotracheal tube

Many institutions, and some older articles written about the process of palliative withdrawal of life supports, have a near-universal practice of removing the patient's oral (or nasal) endotracheal tube. It is generally assumed that patients and families prefer extubation and will be more comfortable after removal of the tube. However, there are some important considerations that may limit or worsen patient comfort after removal of these tubes. Airway compromise caused by edema, trauma, masses, or other lesions may make removal of the oro- or nasoendotracheal tube risky for causing or allowing burdensome symptoms to occur. Similarly, significant hemoptysis or secretions, whether purulent or edematous, may require excessive effort by the patient to clear, and may limit comfort after extubation.

Decades ago, some institutions also routinely removed tracheostomy tubes at end of life. Unless there are specific patient-centered reasons to do so, this is no longer recommended.

4.3 Sedatives, analgesics, anxiolytics

4.3.1 Basal rate titration vs. bolus dose administration

As with enteric opioid medication administration, as needed bolus dose administration and titration should be the mainstay of symptom management. Anecdotally, ICU physicians and nurses often treat opioid and benzodiazepine infusions as though they have the pharmacokinetic and pharmacodynamic properties of vasopressors in terms of time to peak effect and time to steady state. This is not consistent with the actual activity of these medications, and can cause both ineffective symptom management initially, and excessive dosing later in the patient's course.

Pharmacologic principles must be remembered and utilized in the management of infusions of opioids and benzodiazepines. When a patient has significant symptoms, bolus doses can and should be administered as often as the time to peak effect for the drug in question. If the bolus dose is effective in controlling symptoms, the dose can be repeated after time to peak effect when it is needed again. If the dose is only moderately helpful for symptom control, the dose can be increased by 50% at the next administration to improve efficacy. And if the dose is minimally or ineffective, the dose can be doubled at the next dosing interval, or an alternative medication can be considered.

4.3.2 Propofol

Propofol is an anesthetic and sedative without analgesic properties. Some institutions restrict use without a secured airway. However, it can have benefits, including control of seizures, and may occasionally be a helpful adjunct to symptom control for those with severe anxiety, for example, where the patient prefers deep sedation over the possibility of experiencing their severe symptoms at end of life.

4.4 Inhaled vasodilator agents

There are no significant studies to inform best practices on withdrawal of inhaled pulmonary vasodilators. Generally it is probably reasonable to discontinue the agent at the start of transition to comfort measures, before weaning any ventilator settings. Based on half life, symptoms may become significant or severe approximately 15 minutes after discontinuing nitric oxide, or 25 minutes after discontinuing inhaled epoprostenol. Opioid administration as needed for dyspnea or chest pain, and benzodiazepine administration as needed for anxiety after discontinuation are the mainstays of management.

4.5 Neuromuscular blockade agents

Medication must be stopped and effect must be absent prior to withdrawal of life support to ensure ability to demonstrate any discomfort they are experiencing, and to avoid active euthanasia by this mechanism. Even if practicing in a jurisdiction where active euthanasia is legal, withdrawing life support in the presence of neuromuscular blockade is not acceptable because of the temporary and avoidable inability to actively monitor for symptoms and address them during the process.

Ethically, this differs from palliative withdrawal of life support in a neurologically devastated person who is intrinsically unable to demonstrate discomfort during end of life care because their inability to demonstrate discomfort is permanent and irreversible. In this case, for a patient whose surrogate feels the patient would not wish to continue life sustaining treatments, best practice is to aggressively treat for potential symptoms, using changes in vital signs as markers for possible distress and treating accordingly.

Ideally, neuromuscular blockade infusion can be stopped at the initiation of the transition to comfort measures and the effect allowed to wear off gradually as the drug is metabolized. Cessation of neuromuscular blockade allows patients to physically express whether symptoms such as pain, anxiety, dyspnea, or other forms of distress are present.

However, in some instances, patients may have such severe hypoxemia that oxygenation may start to falter before the drug effect is entirely resolved, sometimes to the point that the patient could die before physical symptoms can be fully assessed. In such situations, reversal of neuromuscular blockade may be considered, with neostigmine and glycopyrrolate for any agent, or with sugammadex for rocuronium or vecuronium only.

4.6 Dialysis

When to discontinue dialysis is highly dependent on the patient's situation. For patients with volume overload who are on continuous dialysis, continuing volume removal at least until the time of ventilator withdrawal or extubation may improve comfort by reducing pulmonary edema and whole body anasarca.

For patients with end-stage renal disease, some patients tolerate dialysis well and feel better with continuing it. In the United States, patients who enroll in hospice for a terminal diagnosis not related to their end-stage renal disease may be able to continue outpatient dialysis for a time; this is generally situation-dependent.

4.7 Vasopressors and inotropes

Optimal timing of withdrawal of vasopressors and inotropes is dependent on the situation. For less responsive patients, some physicians recommend discontinuing these early in the course of withdrawal of life supports, to induce a hypotensive or hypoperfusion-related encephalopathy, with the hope of reducing experience of symptoms through this mechanism. Other physicians elect to continue pressors until symptoms are noted to be well controlled after completion of palliative ventilator weaning or withdrawal to ensure medications can be circulated through the body to maximize their effect. Still other physicians discontinue vasopressors and inotropes concurrent with early palliative ventilator withdrawal. To date, there are no studies examining optimal timing; clinical judgment regarding which strategy will most likely meet the individual patient's values, goals, and preferences in light of their condition is needed.

4.8 Pacemakers and implanted cardiac defibrillators

Implanted Cardiac Defibrillators (ICDs) should be deactivated as soon as transition to comfort measures is started, if not already deactivated with DNR order. Implanted pacemakers are typically not deactivated unless the pacemaker function is felt to be significantly prolonging the dying process. Temporary pacemakers are typically deactivated at some point during the withdrawal process; timing can be considered similar to vasopressors.

4.9 Lines, drains, and tubes

At the time of transition to comfort care, the medical team should discuss all lines, drains, and tubes in place and decide whether to maintain or remove each. Urinary catheters may be maintained or removed depending on patient preference and perceived comfort. Temporary central venous catheters and tunneled central venous catheters can generally be maintained unless causing discomfort; temporary catheters may be considered for removal if the patient will be discharged to a setting where use of the catheter may not be feasible.

Nasogastric and orogastric tubes can generally be removed unless continued gastric decompression is necessary or unless there are medications that absolutely must be continued for comfort after extubation. Orogastric tubes should almost always be discontinued if extubation is planned due to significant risk of gagging and oropharyngeal discomfort. Surgical drains and wound vacuum systems should be discussed with the surgical or wound care team.

Pulmonary arterial catheters and arterial lines generally do not improve comfort and should be removed at initiation of transition to comfort measures.

Chest tube management depends on the indication for placement. If a chest tube was initially placed for pneumothorax and maintained in place only because of continued positive pressure ventilation, clamping and removal can be considered, especially if ventilator support will be discontinued. Chest tubes placed for significant, symptomatic pleural effusions likely should be continued to allow continued pleural drainage, unless pleurodesis has occurred. Those placed for pneumothorax that has not resolved likely should also be maintained and kept to suction to avoid symptomatic expansion of the pneumothorax. In all cases, the patient's condition should be the driving factor in decision-making.

4.10 Artificial hydration and nutrition

The limited benefits and significant risks, harms, and symptoms induced by artificial hydration and nutrition should be discussed with the patient or surrogate prior to the palliative withdrawal process. Ideally these should be discontinued hours before initiation of the withdrawal process to avoid full stomachs or fluid overload. Patients who are able to express desire to eat or drink after extubation should be allowed to do so with caution and support, with a focus on comfort and quality of life.

5. Other consideration

5.1 Brain death

Jurisdictions may vary in their laws regarding management of patients diagnosed as brain dead. In some, the local organ procurement organization must be notified and allowed to assess the patient for donation before withdrawal of life supports can be considered.

5.2 Organ and tissue donation

Depending on local or national laws regarding organ and tissue donation, the local organ procurement organization may be required to be notified prior to initiation of the withdrawal process. It may also be required to allow the agency to assess the patient and discuss potential for donation with the patient or surrogate.

Ethically, clinicians involved in the patient's care should not be involved in discussing organ or tissue donation. Perceived or real pressures to procure organs for other patients can adversely affect both decision-making processes of the patient or family and of the medical team. This can also erode the patient's trust in the medical team to prioritize their needs and care. Discussions regarding organ and tissue donation should occur between the patient or family and procurement specialists not involved in the patient's care.

6. Process of palliative ventilator withdrawal

6.1 Time out

Prior to the initiation of palliative withdrawal of life supports, the care team should convene to discuss the patient's condition and formulate a plan consistent with the patient's and family's goals, values, and wishes, and making every effort to minimize or at least control symptoms. This process should be a formal, focused discussion and should occur before initiation in every case. The discussion should include the physician, bedside nurse, and respiratory therapist (RT) at least, ideally should include the chaplain, and the clinical pharmacist when needed.

Topics for discussion during the time out must include plans regarding timing of and method for withdrawing each form of life support, symptoms anticipated due to withdrawal of each life support, and plans for managing these symptoms. The team should also clarify which team member is to be the first point of contact if initial symptom management strategies are insufficient, or if other issues arise.

Where required, the local organ procurement organization must be notified of the plan for palliative withdrawal of life supports and anticipated or possible patient death prior to initiation of the process.

The bedside nurse in particular must be given support and time to focus exclusively or nearly exclusively on the patient undergoing transition to comfort measures, to ensure a smooth transition with excellent symptom management.

Prior to initiation of any steps in the process of withdrawal, the appropriate Do Not Resuscitate order must be signed by the appropriate medical team member. Remaining full code while undergoing palliative withdrawal of life supports is completely counter to the goals of the process; it is absolutely predictable that at some point after withdrawal, cardiopulmonary arrest will occur and require either cessation of efforts based on futility, or require re-initiation of some forms of life support. At best, life supports required at this point might be the same as those in use prior to withdrawal, but more likely would include additional supports to sustain a condition that would at best be equal to the patient's condition at the initiation of withdrawal. If the patient or surrogate desires resuscitative efforts at time of death, current management should be continued. This can include agreed-upon plans to limit escalation (e.g., not adding additional pressors, dialysis, or other new therapies), or to plan to discuss progress, or lack thereof, at a specified date and time, typically a few days.

The patient, surrogate, and family should be asked about what cultural or spiritual practices related to death and dying are meaningful to them, and efforts should be made to support these needs and wishes. These can include Last Rites or specific prayers to be said prior to death, creating memorial items before or after death, and rituals regarding cleaning and care of the patient's body after death. Some memorial items such as handprints, hand casts, recordings, and ECG tracings, can be made fairly easily and inexpensively. Some family members may wish to preserve locks of hair. It is essential to ask open ended questions and not project what the patient or family 'should' or 'should not' want at this point.

Once the plan is created and agreed upon, it should be reviewed with the patient as able, and with the family, to their desired level of detail. Anecdotally, many families and most patients are satisfied hearing that the plan for transition and withdrawal has been discussed and agreed upon by everyone participating, and has been designed to maximize the patient's comfort.

Once transition has started, the bedside nurse should update the designated point of contact for the medical team to discuss any inadequately controlled symptoms or changes in clinical status.

After the patient's death, family should be allowed and encouraged, but never forced, to assist in caring for the patient's body after death. Specific cultural or religious practices regarding care and monitoring of the body after death should be elicited and respected.

7. Case examples

7.1 Case 1: a 'simple' case

Mrs. A is a 78 year-old woman with chronic obstructive lung disease with chronic hypoxic and hypercarbic respiratory failure, and pulmonary cachexia. Her baseline oxygen requirement is 3 liters of oxygen by nasal cannula around the clock. She has been in the intensive care unit (ICU) for three weeks with acute on chronic respiratory failure due to chronic obstructive pulmonary disease (COPD) exacerbation and pneumonia, which have been fully treated. She has failed non-invasive ventilation repeatedly and was reintubated for the third time four days ago. She has spent a total of 16 days on the ventilator thus far. She has mild to moderate secretions and is able to expectorate them without distress. She is on assist control volume control with a tidal volume set at 6 mL/kg ideal body weight, requiring peak inspiratory pressure of 20, rate set at 12, PEEP of 5, and FiO2 35%.

She has a good cuff leak, but failed her spontaneous breathing trial this morning for dyspnea and tachypnea. She requests palliative extubation as she is not amenable to tracheostomy or prolonged ventilatory support.

She is awake, alert, able to write long coherent paragraphs about her understanding of the situation and about her wishes regarding her further care. Her spouse and children are understandably sad but supportive of her wishes, agreeing that this request is consistent with her long-stated wishes regarding prolonged life support. She is on no sedation and reports feeling comfortable on assist control.

After confirming the patient has capacity and is expressing a consistent choice with internally consistent logic based on good understanding of her medical condition, and answering any questions she or her legal surrogate or family have, the physician should discuss with the bedside nurse, RT, and when needed, the ICU charge nurse, to ensure the nurse and RT will have time to properly devote to this patient as the transition to comfort measures occurs. They should discuss what as-needed medications she has been given over her ICU stay, and what her response has been to each, to determine what she is likely to need during the withdrawal process, and orders for these medications should be placed.

The physician or nurse should ask the patient and family if they wish to visit with a chaplain and when. If a chaplain visit is desired prior to transition to comfort measures, the chaplain should ensure they ask about any specific spiritual or cultural practices they wish to observe. If the chaplain's visit is declined, the physician and nurse should coordinate to explore culture or spiritual needs and wishes related to the transition process.

After the appropriate Do Not Resuscitate order is signed, and preparations for symptom management are made, and the patient and family are ready, as she is already on minimal ventilator settings, a spontaneous breathing trial should be initiated again, and comfort medications titrated to maintain her comfort with minimal ventilator support. Once she is comfortable on minimal ventilator support, she can be extubated when she and her family are ready, placed on oxygen via supplemental nasal cannula as is her baseline, and treated with the minimal effective dose of an opioid as needed for pain or dyspnea, or benzodiazepine as needed for primary anxiety, and supported until death or transition to another location for further care.

7.2 Case 2: a more challenging case

Mr. B is a 57 year-old with a remote mid-thoracic spinal cord injury with paraplegia but no known chronic respiratory insufficiency who was admitted to the intensive care unit 2 weeks ago for septic shock due to urinary tract infection with secondary bacteremia. He was initially intubated for respiratory fatigue after hours of working to compensate for lactic acidosis, but developed acute respiratory distress syndrome (ARDS) requiring PEEP of 18 cmH2O at most, FiO2 80–100%, with a set respiratory rate of 34. He has required pressors for the past two weeks, and developed renal failure requiring continuous renal replacement therapy for the past week. He requires deep sedation to maintain ventilator synchrony, and is encephalopathic and agitated when sedation is lightened. When updated at a meeting to discuss his clinical condition and values, preferences, and goals, his legal surrogate states he would not accept prolonged life support measures, including a tracheostomy, a longer-term feeding tube, or more than a few weeks of ventilator support or dialysis. The surrogate feels he has 'had enough' and would not want to continue current management; he feels the patient would wish to have Last Rites administered by a priest, and has no other specific requests for rituals surrounding death.

His code status is changed to Do Not Resuscitate. As soon as is feasible, family and friends are allowed a few hours to visit and say goodbyes. The patient's priest comes to the hospital and administers Last Rites. The patient's nurse and respiratory therapist are relieved of some of their other duties for a time, to be allowed to provide dedicated care to this patient. As discussed in the time out prior to withdrawal, first medications and therapies that do not improve his comfort are discontinued. Renal replacement therapy is then stopped and the machine is removed from the room. Vasopressors are then stopped. Blood pressure falls to a MAP of 50 mmHg but stabilizes, and heart rate increases from 90 to 110 and stabilizes.

His face appears calm and he is synchronous with the ventilator. His current opioid and benzodiazepine infusion rates are continued. Ventilator weaning is initiated; rate is reduced by 4–6 breaths per minute, FiO2 is reduced by 10%, and PEEP by 2 cmH2O simultaneously. Tidal volume is not changed, or may be increased slightly to improve comfort. Any respiratory distress or apparent anxiety are treated with boluses of opioids or benzodiazepines or both, and once controlled, rate, FiO2, and PEEP are weaned again with ongoing boluses and titration of bolus doses as warranted by his symptoms. His SpO2 falls to 60%, but his vital signs remain fairly unchanged. Once he is weaned to 30% with a PEEP of 6, and a set rate of 14 with a total rate of 18, and he appears comfortable based on lack of grimacing and lack of restlessness, the oroendotracheal tube is removed. Additional doses of opioids are given as needed for respiratory discomfort, and benzodiazepines are given as needed for evidence of anxiety. Family remains at the bedside until he dies.

7.3 Case 3: an unusual circumstance

Mr. C is a 30 year-old man with relapsed acute myeloblastic leukemia who develops severe tumor lysis syndrome after induction chemotherapy and is transferred to the ICU for management. He is started on a bicarbonate infusion and IV fluids. He is placed on BiPAP to support his respiratory compensation for acidemia while arrangements are made to start continuous renal replacement therapy, but is unable to maintain respiratory compensation for acidemia and is intubated. His respiratory rate is moderate, with minimal pressure and oxygen requirements. He remains remarkably alert, calm, and coherent after medications given for intubation wear off. After discussion of his overall condition, in which he has fully participated, he writes out clearly that he wants to transition to comfort care. The medical team discusses his physiologic derangements and recalls his extremely high respiratory rate prior to initiation of bicarbonate infusion. After a short spontaneous breathing trial in which he remains somewhat tachypneic but does not feel distressed.

He requests his code status be changed to Do Not Resuscitate and Do Not Intubate; these orders are completed. He is extubated to allow him to speak with his family. Continuous renal replacement therapy is continued for a few more hours until the cassette requires changing, at which time the set-up is taken down and not restarted. Bicarbonate infusion is continued to ameliorate his acidemia in hope of preventing dyspnea due to tachypnea. He is offered opioids for dyspnea when he appears to have respiratory distress and allowed to choose whether or not he feels he needs them, as well as being allowed to request them when needed. After several hours of good conversations with his family, he feels his breathing is tiring out and requests more frequent opioids, even if this means he may be too sleepy to interact with family. Opioids are given to relieve his dyspnea and respiratory distress. When the bicarbonate infusion bag is nearly empty, the rate is reduced and opioids are titrated to comfort before the bag is completed and the infusion stopped. His breathing pattern becomes irregula as he is no longer able to maintain compensation, and he appears comfortable until and through his death.

7.4 Case 4: a very challenging case

Mx. D is a 37 year-old person with antiphospholipid antibody syndrome and patent foramen ovale, with multiple deep venous thromboses and pulmonary emboli in the past, on therapeutic anticoagulation, develops diffuse alveolar hemorrhage and acute hypoxic respiratory failure requiring intubation and mechanical ventilation. They are treated with steroids and inhaled tranexamic acid, and chronic anticoagulation is held. They unfortunately have several seizures and are found to have multiple embolic strokes with severe hemorrhagic conversion, including several of the cerebellum and visual cortex. On meeting with their family including parents who are their legal surrogate, they feel that the likely long-term impairments caused by the strokes would be unacceptable given their career as a dancer, and that they would not want to continue disease-directed therapies.

Given the continued moderate and occasionally large volume hemoptysis requiring suctioning through the oroendotracheal tube, the patient's sibling, who is a respiratory therapist, expresses concern about the patient's ability to breathe comfortably if extubated. Code status is changed to Do Not Resuscitate prior to transition to comfort care. Ventilator support is weaned down to the lowest PEEP level at which the patient appears comfortable. Pressure support, SIMV-PSV, and APRV with only a small difference between high and low PEEP. The medical team advises their family that the ventilator will continue to trigger after the patient's death, as the ventilator's apnea backup settings can be minimized but not completely discontinued. Their comfort is maintained with opioid and benzodiazepines as needed until death.

7.5 Case 5: organ procurement

Ms. E is a 25 year-old woman with a long-standing history of opioid abuse including ingestion and injection- both subcutaneous and intravenous- of prescription opioid pills, and injection of heroin and fentanyl. She has suffered several overdoses requiring hospitalization and brief periods of intubation and mechanical ventilation in the past, has undergone rehab including some periods of abstinence, but has unfortunately suffered multiple relapses. Five days ago she was found unresponsive with agonal breathing at home after last speaking to family by phone hours earlier. MRI of the brain and serial head CT scans over several days in the ICU showed diffuse anoxic injury with severe edema and progressive herniation. Her clinical exam with normal electrolytes, normal temperature, and normal pCO2 and pH progresses to demonstrate no brainstem reflexes.

Several forms of testing clearly demonstrate brain death. The medical team informs and consoles her family, and requests the chaplain and social worker to further assist in supporting the family. The bedside nurse contacts the local organ procurement organization, whose representative comes to the hospital and reviews Ms. E's case. She is noted to be a self-registered organ donor, and is deemed to be a candidate for donation of multiple organs. The representative from the organ procurement organization discusses with her family the process of assessing her and preparing for potential organ donation. She is maintained on mechanical ventilation via oroendotracheal tube. Pituitary failure is managed with IV levothyroxine, DDAVP, and hydrocortisone. Blood pressure is maintained with vasopressors. When assessment is complete and the organ procurement organization and explant surgeons are available, she is taken to the operating room with a solemn procession in her honor, where life supports are withdrawn simultaneously. Cardiac death occurs 20 minutes later, and all viable organs are harvested for transplantation.

8. Conclusions

The above discussions, and the case examples, are not exhaustive of the situations clinicians may find themselves facing in the course of caring for patients. They are examples of some of the more common conditions that require consideration and flexibility for patient-centered management. Far from a simple, 'one size fits all' process, they illustrate that palliative withdrawal of life supports is a medical procedure that requires thoughtful collaboration and consideration to provide each patient with the most comfortable transition to end of life care possible.

Author details

Lauren F. Goodman
Department of Internal Medicine, Division of Pulmonary, Critical Care, and Sleep Medicine, The Ohio State University Wexner Medical Center, The Ohio State University College of Medicine, Columbus, Ohio, USA

*Address all correspondence to: lauren.goodman@osumc.edu